Ketogenic Diet for Beginners

How to Slim Down and Burn Fat, Highly Effective Step by Step 30 Day Keto Program for Women and Men with Bonus Intermittent Fasting Content for Ultimate Weight Loss

Christine Moore

© Copyright 2019 - All rights reserved.

The content contained within this book may not be reproduced, duplicated or transmitted without direct written permission from the author or the publisher.

Under no circumstances will any blame or legal responsibility be held against the publisher, or author, for any damages, reparation, or monetary loss due to the information contained within this book. Either directly or indirectly.

Legal Notice:
This book is copyright protected. This book is only for personal use. You cannot amend, distribute, sell, use, quote or paraphrase any part, or the content within this book, without the consent of the author or publisher.

Disclaimer Notice:
Please note the information contained within this document is for educational and entertainment purposes only. All effort has been executed to present accurate, up to date, and reliable, complete information. No warranties of any kind are declared or implied. Readers acknowledge that the author is not engaging in the rendering of legal, financial, medical or professional advice. The content within this book has been derived from various sources. Please consult a licensed professional before attempting any techniques outlined in this book.

By reading this document, the reader agrees that under no circumstances is the author responsible for any losses, direct or indirect, which are incurred as a result of the use of information contained within this document, including, but not limited to, — errors, omissions, or inaccuracies.

Contents

Introduction _____ 1

Chapter 1:
The Basics of the Ketogenic Diet _____ 3

Chapter 2:
The Benefits of the Ketogenic Diet _____ 14

Chapter 3:
Why the Keto Diet is Popular _____ 21

Chapter 4:
The Ultimate Ketogenic Shopping List _____ 25

Chapter 5:
Shopping List Summary _____ 37

Chapter 6:
Greater Keto Success with Clean Eating _____ 42

Chapter 7:
Meal Prepping on the Keto Diet _____ 58

Chapter 8:
Meal Prep Basics Recap _____ 72

Chapter 9:
The Principles of the Ketogenic Reset Diet _____ 86

Chapter 10:
The Keto Diet and Intermittent Fasting _____ 88

Chapter 11:
The 30-Day Ketogenic Diet Plan for Success _____ 92

Chapter 12:
Delicious Ketogenic Recipes to Try! _____ 99

Chapter 13:
Ketogenic Tips and Tricks _____ 139

Conclusion _____ 144

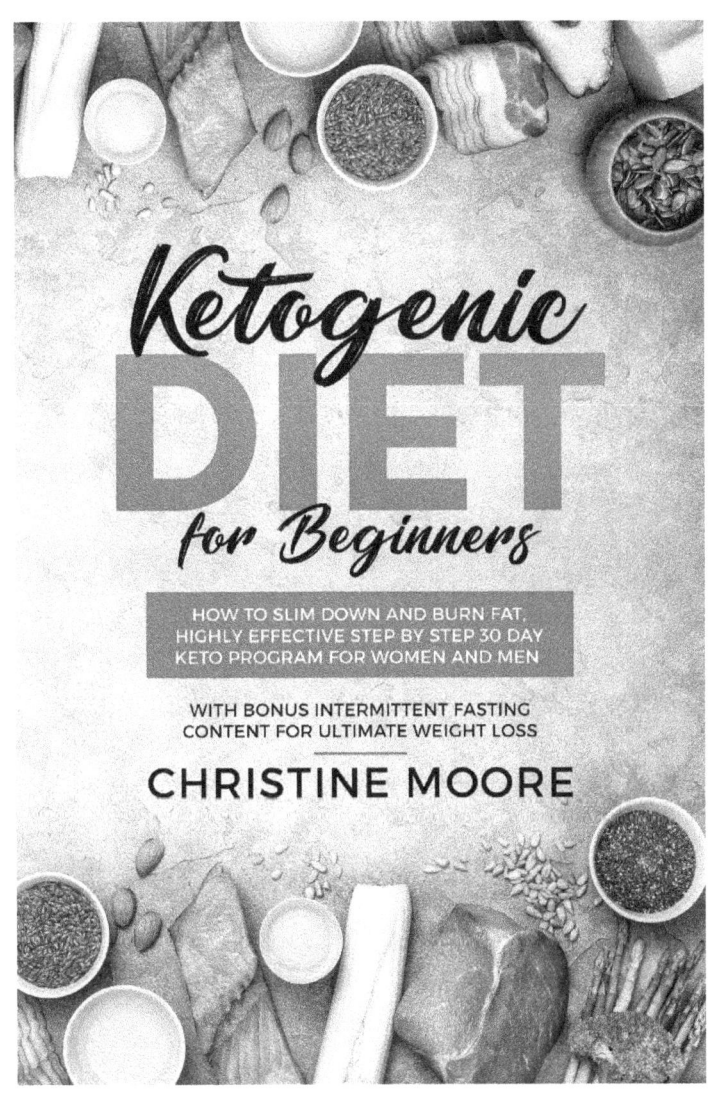

Introduction

Thanks to all the convenience of the 21st century, many people are devouring junk without even realizing it. The freezer aisles and fast food places have become the cornerstone of our nutrition, which is leaving thousands of people overindulging on excess sugars, sodium, and carbohydrates.

So, where does one turn when there are equally as many diets that claim it can help anyone lose weight by eating magical bars and powders? The overload of information is certainly enough to confuse and stress out those that simply want to lose weight and feel better about themselves mentally and physically.

Thankfully, not all diets are created equally negative. Unlike other low-carb diets, this book will introduce and educate you on the in-depth basics of the Ketogenic Diet; a diet that enables your body to fuel itself from fats instead of carbohydrates.

I know what you are thinking: Fats? Aren't fats *bad* for you?! Sure, they can be. But only when you gorge on trans and saturated fats. When eaten correctly, the consumption of healthy fats kick-starts your body and puts it into ketosis, which enables a faster rate of weight loss while feeling great! A win-win for everyone!

There are many books on the Ketogenic Diet, but none are quite as thorough as this one. Within this book, you will learn:

- The basics of the Ketogenic Diet
- Keto benefits
- How to intertwine the Keto Diet with intermittent fasting
- How to use meal prepping to ensure your ketogenic success
- A 30-day plan and delicious sample recipes to get yourself on the right track
- And much more!

Chapter 1:
The Basics of the Ketogenic Diet

The Ketogenic Diet is not just a diet, but a large part of an entire change to your overall lifestyle. There are millions of people that have taken the Keto Diet seriously and experienced amazing results. Whether you believe it or not, I know you have the power within you to make this healthy change, too!

Instead of using excuses and placing roadblocks in your way, you do have what it takes to look great as you devour delicious and natural foods that will benefit both your mental and physical health and give you the energy to take life by the horns!

Of course, to be successful on any diet, you will need to understand the basics of how the human body functions and how diets effect your physical wellbeing.

There is an array of low-calorie, gluten-free, and low-fat diets out there. I have no doubt that you have heard of South Beach, Weight Watches, Atkins, and the hundreds of other similar diet fads. What do all these diets have in common? They make you starve yourself as you try to stomach bland foods and push through phases of induction.

It is not rocket science; these diets are not all nutritionally sound and can make you feel worse than you were when you were hitting the drive-thru every day. These are not sustainable and cannot become a part of your long-term lifestyle.

So, what do the better and more successful diets that people talk about have in common? Simple, a *reduction of foods that are high in carbohydrates*. It has been scientifically proven that low-carb diets help reduce weight with the consumption of fewer calories than that of low-fat diets. These dieters also have improved insulin and blood sugar levels, as well as triglyceride numbers.

If have purchased this book with not one clue as to what the Ketogenic Diet is, there is no need to fret. We will discuss the details about the crucial aspects as to what has made this diet so popular.

What is the Ketogenic Diet?

Before we dive in, you can rest assured that this diet does not shackle you with the task of counting calories. It simply is centered around the consumption of devouring a diet this is low in carbohydrates and high in fat.

- "What? High in fat? Isn't eating too much fat terrible for your body?"

You would naturally think this because that is what we have been taught to believe since we were wee tots! But the ketogenic diet stems directly from the natural process known as 'ketosis' that gives our bodies the opportunity to thrive when our intake of food is lowered.

The phrase 'ketogenic' is stemmed from the natural process of 'ketosis', which allows our bodies to thrive when the intake of food might be low. Ketones are produced during this process as fats in our livers break down. The entire goal of the ketogenic diet is to force our bodies to stay within this state of high metabolism.

No, it is not about starving yourself and keeping yourself from consuming food, but rather the starvation of consuming carbohydrates. Humans have not changed in the fact that we can adapt to our environments at drastic speeds. When you pack your body with bad edibles, it will start to burn those precious ketones that are partially responsible for weight loss and optimum mental and physical performance.

How the Keto Came to Be

Weirdly enough, the ketogenic diet has been around for quite a few decades. It was developed by a guy named Dr. Russell Wilder back in the year 1924. It was quite the concoction that treated epilepsy but unfortunately fell through due to the creation of anti-seizure medications that came about during the 1940's. It didn't make much of an appearance until the mid-1990's, when the Abraham family began the Charlie Foundation for their son, Charlie. Charlie's body did not handle all that anti-seizure pill-popping very well. He began following the means of the ketogenic diet as a toddler and stuck to it for a time period of five years. He is now a successful college student and is still to this day seizure-free.

The bottom line is that the ketogenic diet is made up of extremely low-carb and high-fat intakes. This diet is quite like that of the Atkins and other low-carb diets. While you are reducing your intake of carbohydrates by such drastic amounts, you are replacing it with foods high in fat.

The absence of carbs creates a highly metabolic state within your body, known as ketosis (as mentioned above.) In Layman's terms, our body becomes an incredibly powered working machine, burning off fat for energy instead of ketones. It warps our metabolisms so that it no longer burns precious substances utilized to keep our bodies in the best shape they can be.

This diet has been shown to reduce blood sugars and insulin levels, which makes it a diet that is loaded with quite a few health benefits. You will read about some of these benefits later in this chapter.

The Fundamentals of Ketosis

When your body is in a ketosis state, your liver creates ketones which then are your body's main source of energy. The core of the ketogenic diet is based on the idea that our bodies were made to run better as a *fat burner* rather than a burner of sugar and carbs for energy. The ketogenic diet reverses the way in which your body functions in a positive manner. This means it has the power to totally change your perspective of healthy nutrition!

The primary goal of maintaining ketosis on the ketogenic diet is to force your body to a metabolic state. You do not want to do this through starvation, but rather through the starvation of carbohydrates. Our bodies are very adaptable, so when you switch your diet by loading it with fats instead of carbs, your body begins to burn off the ketones as an energy source. When you get to burning off optimal ketone levels, you then can lose weight faster, feel better, and personally experience the physical and mental performance benefits the ketogenic diet has to offer.

The ketogenic diet is made up of extremely low-carb and high-fat intakes. This diet is like the Atkins diet and other low-carb diets. While you are reducing your intake of carbohydrates by such drastic amounts, you are replacing it with foods with a high fat content. By doing this, you trick your metabolism so that it no longer burns precious substances utilized to keep our bodies in the best shape they can be.

How Ketosis Works

Ketosis is a form of acidosis, which means it disrupts the pH balance in the body, due to the presence of more ketones in the blood. Ketones are a by-product of metabolizing fat and are released when the fat consumed is broken down into an energy source.

Metabolism on ketosis is when blood sugars are not readily available to your body for a source of energy, your body switches gears and starts to break down fat instead. When the ketones are broken down from glucose and released into the bloodstream, this is the start of ketosis. Produced in the liver, ketones can be utilized for other metabolic processes in the body.

Reaching a State of Ketosis

Getting your body into a ketosis state may seem complex to those that are brand new to the whole ketogenic concept. But it is a very simple process once you get the hang of it:

Restricting carbs. Many people tend to focus on their consumption of net carbs when they should be limiting total carbs. Try your best to stay below 20g of net carbs and 35g of total carbs.

Restricting protein consumption. Beginners on the keto have a knack for forgetting their intake of protein. Eating too much protein can lead to drastically low levels of ketosis. For weight loss, you want to eat around 0.6-0.8 grams per pound to achieve that lean body mass.

Don't fret over fat. Fat is the primary source of energy on the keto diet, so you need to make it a priority to fuel your body with enough of it.

Drink plenty of water: This is especially vital when you first begin the keto diet! Make it a goal to need to stay hydrated to regulate your bodily functions and control your levels of hunger.

Quit reaching for snacks: You can lose weight much easier when your body doesn't undergo multiple spikes in insulin throughout the day. Snacking for no reason will lessen your weight loss achievements.

Fast: Fasting is a good tool to help in the boosting of ketone levels. Different ideas of fasting include: skipping a meal, condense your intake of food to a 4 to 7-hour window and leave the remaining time to fast, or 24 to 48-hour cleanses involve not eating for 1 to 2 days to experience extended fasting periods.

Incorporate exercise: Exercise is a healthy habit for everyone. If you want to get the most out of undergoing the ketogenic diet, add 20 to 30 minutes or more of regular exercise each day. Even an extra walk can help regulate blood sugar and promote more weight loss.

Take supplements: While this is not necessary, it can allow you to achieve what you want from the keto diet easier.

How to Know When Your Body Reaches Ketosis

There are many resources that you will come across in your hunt for figuring out how to achieve optimal ketosis. Trash all those and listen up! The best ketosis can be achieved through diet and nutrition alone! There is no magic pill, shortcut, or gimmick that will help you reach it.

There is one method of measuring your ketone levels that involves you urinate on a strip of paper, but these can be inaccurate and can cost loads of money. Instead, know the physical symptoms that will naturally tell you that you are on the right track:

Increased urination: The ketogenic diet is a natural diuretic that increases acetoacetate, a ketone body that is excreted through the process of urinating.

Dry mouth: When you urinate more often, you are naturally going to have a drier mouth and be thirstier much more frequently. This is another reason to drink lots of water so that you replenish your electrolytes effectively.

Bad breath: A ketone body known as acetone is excreted into our mouth which effects the smell of our breath. It tends to smell like ripe fruit, sometimes even as potent as nail polish remover. This is temporary and goes away over time.

Reduced hunger and increased energy: After you get past the "keto flu" stage, you will experience much high energy levels, a clear state of mind and you are hungry less often.

Ketoacidosis

I hear all the time about the confusion that ketogenic beginners have about the difference between ketosis and ketoacidosis. Ketoacidosis occurs in people who are diabetic and is a complication of type 1 diabetes. This happens when high levels of ketones are in blood sugars and can be life-threatening. It makes your blood acidic, which can risk the functioning of your vital organs.

Burning Sugar Vs. Burning Fat

When you eat foods that are high in carb count, such as that delicious breakfast donut, your body must make glucose and insulin to break it down properly:

- Glucose is an easily converted molecule that is converted by the body into a source of energy

- Insulin is made to help process the glucose that hits your bloodstream when you eat that donut.

Fats are not needed by the body when it has glucose as a primary energy source. This means fat is stored, which is what contributes to that excess weight that you hate carrying around. When your body utilizes all the glucose, your brain signals your body to reach for a snack, which often for most is unhealthy.

Therefore, the ketogenic diet has the power to completely reverse the effects of eating unhealthy by switching the source of energy that your body picks to burn. When you lessen your consumption of carbs and sugar, your body then must find another source of energy, which is when your body enters a ketosis state.

When your body is in ketosis, fat cells release any water stored and the fat cells can enter the bloodstream and head to the liver. This is the main goal of the keto diet. Despite popular belief, you cannot enter ketosis by starving your body, but rather by starving yourself of consuming carbohydrates. It is essential to know this crucial difference.

Different Types of the Ketogenic Diet

Just like other diets, there are a few variations of the ketogenic diet that you must choose from depending on your needs, wants, and goals:

High-protein keto diet is made up of all the ketogenic basics but allows you to eat more protein. It is made up of 5 percent carbs, 35 percent protein, and 60 percent fat.

Targeted keto diet is a version that allows you to add the consumption of carbs according to your workout times for more energy.

Cyclical keto diet is a version that allows you to incorporate periods of high carb refeeds. For instance, you eat strictly keto for 5 days and then eat foods that are higher in carbohydrates for 2 days.

Standard keto diet is the basic version of the keto diet where you are supposed to eat foods that are high in fat content and low in carb count while consuming large amounts of protein. It is made up of 5 percent carbs, 20 percent protein, and 75 percent fat.

Out of all the versions, standard keto and the high-protein versions are the only ones that have been extensively studied. The targeted and cyclical versions are more advanced and are typically used by athletes and/or bodybuilders only. The information within this book will focus on the standard ketogenic, for it is the most recommended and has been found to be far more successful in everyday individuals.

Importance of 'Macros'

Macros is the abbreviation for *macronutrients*. These nutrients are made up of the "big 3", known as carbohydrates, protein, and fats.

Fats are 10 percent anti-ketogenic and 90 percent ketogenic, thanks to the small amount of glucose that is released as our bodies convert the triglycerides.

Proteins are 58 percent anti-ketogenic and 46 percent ketogenic because insulin levels rise from half of the proteins, we ingest that are converted to glucose.

Carbs are 100 percent anti-ketogenic since they are responsible for the rise in insulin and blood glucose levels.

What does this mean? That carbs and protein will lessen your body's ability to get into the state of ketosis. It's vital to learn how they are being converted to energy, which is through the metabolic pathways after being ingested as nutrients.

Your Body and the Ketogenic Diet

I have no doubt that with all this newfound information that you are likely curious to how you will be feeling when you first start undergoing the keto transformation.

Your body is more than likely accustomed to a simple routine of breaking down the carbohydrates you consume into energy. Your body has already built up the enzymes it needs to process these carbs, which means they are by no means used to dealing with the breaking down and storage of fats.

Your body must become used to the lack of glucose it is being provided and deal with the increase in fat, which makes the creation of brand-new enzymes. Once your body starts to become used to the state of ketosis, you will naturally shift to utilize what glucose you have left in storage. As a result, your muscles will have a depleted supply of glycogen, which can mean lethargy and a lack of overall energy.

The first week of undergoing the keto diet, many people report being dizzy, easily aggravated, and have headaches. This is because your electrolytes are being flushed from your system. Another reason why you must drink lots of water and keep up with a sodium intake. In fact, it is said by professionals to go overboard with the salt you consume, because it helps you retain more water, which replenishes your electrolytes.

Chapter 2:
The Benefits of the Ketogenic Diet

Low-carb diets have been a subject for controversy for years. It has been said that diets high in fat content would raise cholesterol levels through the roof, causing heart disease and other bad body ailments. But research has been changing the face of low-carb dieting.

Despite the controversy, low-carb diets are the ones that have won the race against other diets when it comes to scientific tests. They are not only a great substitute when trying to lose weight, but they even have other great health benefits, even reducing cholesterol levels.

Benefits of the Keto Diet

The main component that is largely working in your body during your time on the ketogenic diet is the process of ketosis. Creating this metabolic state has been proven to have drastically positive effects, even if only on the diet for a short time. Here are some grand benefits of ketosis itself first!

- Increases our body's capabilities to use fats as a source of fuel.

- Ketosis has a protein-sparing effect, which means our bodies prefer utilizing ketones as opposed to glucose.

- Lowers levels of insulin within our bodies, which contains a lipolysis-blocking effect, which reduces the utilization of fatty acids as a source of energy. When insulin levels are lowered, growth hormones and other growth factors can then be released without an issue.

Suppresses Hunger

Naturally, many diets require you to eat less than your body is used to. Because of this, never-ending hunger pains always seem to strike and at the worst times. This is the main reason people tend to feel miserable while on any diet plan. Diets that are low in carb intake are great because it automatically reduces your appetite. Those who cut carbs and consume more proteins and fat eat *fewer* calories.

More Potential for Weight Loss

It doesn't take a scientist to know that reducing several carbs we consume will directly contribute to weight loss. People who stick within the means of low-carb diets lose weight at a much faster rate than those who within the means of a low-carb diet. Diets low in carbohydrates tend to help in the reduction of excess water in our bodies, which can add on the pounds. The ketogenic diet reduces insulin levels too, meaning the kidneys are shedding all that excess sodium that can lead to retaining extra weight.

Reduction of Triglycerides

That long term is a fancy name for fat molecules. These little boogers contribute to ailments such as heart disease. When people reduce the consumption of carbs, there is quite a lessening of triglycerides building up in our bodies.

Increase Good Cholesterol Levels

(HDL) is the kind of cholesterol you *want* to have. The ketogenic diet helps with raising the levels of HDL because of the consumption of fats. There are major bodily improvements when the levels of good and bad cholesterol start to shift.

Reduces Blood Sugar and Insulin Levels

When we consume carbs, they are broken into simple sugars by our digestive system. They then go into our blood streams and elevate blood sugar levels. High sugars can be toxic, which is why insulin exists. There are many people who have a type of diabetes not only because of blood lines and genetics but because they have not eaten the best for quite a bit of their life. Their bodies no longer recognize insulin when it is attempting to help lower blood sugar levels. With the ketogenic diet, it has been seen that blood sugar and insulin levels come way down.

Reduction in Blood Pressure

Diets that are low in carbohydrates are effective in reducing blood pressure levels, which can assist us in living longer. When blood pressure is high, we are at greater risks of developing hypertension and other ailments.

Natural Treatment for Cancer

Properly regulating your bodies metabolic functions has been proven to be a great step in reducing and even treating cancer. Reducing or totally removing carbs from your diet can help in the deletion of energy from cancerous cells and stop them from spreading.

Effective in Treating Metabolic Syndrome

This syndrome is a serious medical condition that is associated with heart disease and diabetes. There are several symptoms:

- Low levels of HDL
- High triglyceride levels
- Raised fasting blood sugar levels
- Elevated blood pressure
- Abdominal obesity

The best news? Incorporating a low-carb diet into your life can drastically reduce all these symptoms. The ketogenic diet has the key to unlock a much healthier physical life.

Therapy for Some Brain Disorders

There are certain areas of our brains that strictly run on glucose as a fuel. This is the reason behind why our livers produce it from protein if we do not consume carbs. There are bigger portions of our brains, however, that burn through ketones.

In studies, more than half of children who utilized the ketogenic diet had a 50% reduction in seizures. This diet, among other low-carb diets, are being studied as to what its effect is on brain disorders like Parkinson's and Alzheimer's disease.

Risks of the Keto Diet

Just like with every good thing in the world, there are some risk factors to consider before diving headfirst on your journey with the ketogenic diet.

The Keto Flu

This type of flu is a common phenomenon for newbies on the ketogenic diet, but thankfully it goes away just after a few days. You might experience mild discomfort in the form of cramps, nausea, headaches, and fatigue. The keto flu happens thanks to two main reasons:

- You are going to the bathroom more often to urinate, which means you are losing electrolytes and water within the body. You can combat this easily by drinking Powerade Zero or a bouillon cube in water.

- Your body is in a phase of total transition. You are used to processing a higher intake of carbohydrates. Your body needs a bit of time to create the enzymes needed to process a higher intake of fat. Therefore, you may feel low on energy. It is best to gradually decrease your intake of carbs and not go cold turkey.

- Once you increase your water consumption and replace electrolytes, you will find the symptoms of the keto flu to decrease or totally diminish. For a person that is beginning the transition to the ketogenic diet, its recommended to eat less than 15 grams of carbs a day and decrease over time.

Fatigue and Irritability

Even though raised ketone levels can drastically improve a few areas regarding your physical quality of life, they are also directly related to feeling tired and having to work harder during physical activities.

Brain Fog

If you stay on the ketogenic diet long term, there is going to be some major shifting when it comes to the metabolic areas of the body. This can make you moody and somewhat sluggish, which can make you not able to think clearly or adequately focus. Ensure that you are reducing your levels of carb intake at steady levels, not all at once.

Lipids May Change

Even though fats on the ketogenic diet are welcomed, if you consume large amounts of saturated fats, your cholesterol levels will begin to increase. Make sure you are consuming healthy fats.

Micronutrient Deficiencies

Diets that consist of low-carb foods are more than likely lacking in essential nutrients, such as magnesium, potassium, and iron. You might want to strongly consider finding a high-quality multivitamin to take daily.

The Possibility of Developing Ketoacidosis

If your ketone levels become too wacky, it may lead to this condition. pH levels within your blood decrease, creating an environment that is high in acidity, which can be threatening for those with diabetes.

Muscle Loss

As you consume less energy, your body leans on the help of other tissues as a source of fuel. When working out heavily while on a diet like the ketogenic, there is the potential for major muscle loss.

Chapter 3:
Why the Keto Diet is Popular

Unless you have been stuck under a rock, most of the world knows at least a little something about the Ketogenic Diet and how it can help your body become shaped into its peak condition.

The Ketogenic Diet was first introduced as a legit method to treat children with epilepsy, which it is still famous for today. However, it went into remission for decades until 1994, after a Mr. Jim Abrahams started the *Charlie Foundation*, thanks to his son who was helped by this magical diet that ended his days of life-altering seizures.

Since 1994, the foundation has helped grow educational resources for that that want to learn more about the diet and possibly start it for themselves. Then, Quest Nutrition, a company that was created to harness the popularity of the diet, started to study the effects the keto diet had on the body's metabolism. So, why is the Ketogenic Diet so dang popular? Here are a few reasons.

We as humans enjoy breaking the food pyramid's standards Let's face it; the food pyramid we learned in school is broken and nothing like it used to be. It is totally wrong and not really working. We have been taught to eat certain ways and while many of us try our best to stick to those lessons, we still fail. The Ketogenic Diet helps us to recreate the idea of the food pyramid. The keto pyramid looks completely different:

- The bottom portion is filled with nutrient dense nuts, healthy fats, and antioxidant herbs

- The next portion is loaded with proteins high in quality and meats that are marbled with healthy fats

- The next portion has bright vegetables with natural low-sugar nutrients.

- The top portion is small but has room for naturally sweet foods, for fruits and ketogenic-approved treats.

We are Sick of Fighting with Our Bodies

The Ketogenic Diet is appealing to hundreds of people since it is directly parallel to how our bodies thrive naturally. Not very many folks choose the right things to eat when they are having cravings and really want to eat something else.

From personal experience, when I was on the keto diet, I very seldom had negative cravings. When your body is in ketosis, living and eating are simplified, and your body naturally feels happier. You feel good, which makes total sense because eating a keto diet:

- Decreases hunger which results in weight loss

- Improves overall brain function

- Helps with gut health

- Decreases blood pressure

- Stabilizes insulin in the body

Simply, the ketogenic diet allows your body to work the way it was naturally designed, and you don't feel like you are constantly losing a battle with yourself.

The Ketogenic Diet is super big right now because it honestly just makes *sense*. It has been everyday people as well as famous folks the results they want. It is a diet that they can stick with long-term because they no longer feel deprived, which is the secret for why it has worked for so many people!

Paleo vs. Ketogenic

Along with the popularity of the Ketogenic Diet came the Paleo Diet, a tribute to our caveman ancestors. But the rise of the caveman way of life was a short-lived fad compared to the keto diet for multiple reasons:

- No one is researching the Paleo Diet these days. Google knows when something is popular and the charts in 2018 do not lie. Between 2010 and 2017 was the prime time for the Paleo Diet, but in 2018, it dropped to 27% popularity.

- Enthusiasts who thrived on the Paleo Diet have since sold themselves out. The paleo at the beginning was revolutionary, changing the course of how people fueled their body. Now, the companies and influencers who sell ready-made paleo "junk" is what the paleo seems to be about.

- The packaged paleo meals that are ready to eat are just about as bad as stuffing your face with a pack of Oreos. Cooking "lovely and lightly" is very ironic, since it requires people to microwave meals, which is something the "paleo lifestylists" dislike doing.

The Paleo Diet fad, despite how hard people tried to get it accurate, was historically inaccurate and difficult to follow. The quantities of meat, veggies, and fruits that we consume today cannot resemble what our Paleolithic ancestors ate. Kale, broccoli, and cauliflower were not existent back then, and dairy and grains are forbidden on the diet, even though grains technically did exist.

Chapter 4:
The Ultimate Ketogenic Shopping List

To be successful while undergoing any diet, you need to know what to devour and what to avoid. In this chapter, we will cover this in detail!

Ketogenic Diet Foods Groups
All the below food groups can adhere to the strict 5 percent allowance of carbohydrates that you can consume on the keto diet.

- *Fats and oils:* the more natural, the better. Do your best to get fats and oils from nuts and meats. Supplement your diet with saturated and monounsaturated fats such as olive oil, butter, and coconut oil

- *Protein:* grab grass-fed, pasture-raised, or organic meats when you can

- *Vegetables:* doesn't matter if you choose from fresh or frozen. Lean towards above ground veggies, especially leafy greens.

- *Dairy:* most dairy is perfectly fine to eat on the keto, but ensure you are purchasing full-fat items, for they tend to have fewer carbs.

- *Nuts and Seeds:* nuts and seeds in moderation can be used to create meals with delicious textures! The fattier the nuts, such as almonds and macadamia, the better.

- *Beverages:* do your best to stick to drinking water. Feel free to flavor your water with lemon and lime juice or other stevia-based flavorings

Fats and Oils

As you have already learned, fats are going to be taking up the majority of what you devour while you are on the ketogenic diet, which means you need to make choices based around your likes and dislikes. You can combine them in various ways, such as topping your meat with butter, or in sauces and dressings. There are different kinds of fats that are involved with a healthy balance on the keto diet. Various foods have different combinations of fats, but you need to ensure you are avoiding unhealthy fats.

- Saturated fats are good for you, this includes lard, butter, ghee, coconut oil, etc.

- Monounsaturated fats are great on the keto diet, this includes macadamia nuts and oils, avocado, olive, olive oils, etc.

- Polyunsaturated fats are in fatty fish and animal proteins and should be incorporated into your keto diet. However, processed polyunsaturated fats are bad for you and are found in items such as margarine.

- Trans fats should always be avoiding. They are heavily processed and chemically altered to lengthen their shelf live. Avoid hydrogenated fat items; they are linked to heart disease.

- Monounsaturated and saturated fats, such as egg yolks, coconut oil, avocado, macadamia nuts, and butter are stable chemically and are less inflammatory.

Ideal Ketogenic Fats and Oils:

- Avocado oil
- Avocados
- Butter or ghee
- Cocoa butter
- Coconut butter
- Coconut oil
- Egg yolks
- Fatty fishes
- Macadamia and Brazil nuts
- Macadamia nut oil
- Mayonnaise
- MCT oil
- Non-hydrogenated animal fat
- Olive oil
- Tallow

Protein

The best bet you can make when incorporating more protein into your ketogenic diet are grass-fed or pasture-raised options. This lessens the bacteria and steroid hormones you will be consuming. Choose darker meats when you can with poultry since darker poultry is fattier than white meat. And feel free to eat lots of healthy fatty fish. They are great in omega-3's.

When choosing red meats, there is not much you must avoid. Cured meats and sausages tend to have added processed ingredients and additional sugars. If you consume steak, lean towards fattier cuts, such as ribeye. If you like to devour hamburger meat, try to choose fat ratios such as 85/15 or 80/20.

When dealing with protein on the ketogenic diet, you need to be aware of how much you are consuming; eating too much protein can lead to lower ketosis levels and an increase in glucose production. Try to balance your protein between meals with fattier sauces and side dishes. If you opt for a leaner beef, you need to be careful about portioning it as protein. Jerky and other beefy snacks can enable your total consupmption of protein to add up rather quickly, so ensure you pair it with cheese or something else fatty!

- Fish (Preferably wild-caught; the fattier, the better): catfish, cod, flounder, halibut, mackerel, mahi-mahi, salmon, snapper, trout, and tuna.

- Shellfish: Squid, mussels, scallops, crab, lobster, oysters, clams.

- Whole eggs: Purchase free-range eggs from local markets. You can prepare them scrambled, poached, boiled, deviled, and yes, even fried!

- Beef: Ground beef, stew meat, roasts, steaks. The fattier, the better.

- Pork: Ham, tenderloin, pork chops, pork loin, ground pork.

- Poultry: Pheasant, quail, duck, chicken, other wild game.

- Organs: Tongue, kidney, liver, heart, offal.

- Other proteins: Turkey, lamb, goat, veal, other wild game.

- Bacon and sausage: Check labels to ensure your choices are not cured with sugar or have additional fillers. Don't worry yourself with nitrates.

- Nut butters: Opt for natural and unsweetened nuts and lean towards the fattier versions of macadamia nut and almond butters.

Fruits and Vegetables

Veggies are a grand portion of a healthy and well-balanced ketogenic diet. But you still must be aware, however, since many vegetables are high in sugar and just don't make the nutritional cut. The best veggies on the keto diet are ones high in nutrients and low in carbs. As you can imagine, the darker and leafier, the better! If a veggie closely resembles spinach or kale, then you are on the right track.

Lean towards cruciferous veggies that grow above the ground and that are green and leafy. If you want to consume fewer pesticide residues, then purchase organic, but this is not necessary for the ketogenic diet to work for you. In fact, both organic and non-organic fruits and veggies have the exact same nutritional qualities. Fresh or frozen are both great options!

Veggies that grow below the ground can still be enjoyed on the keto diet but need to be heavily moderated since they are loaded with natural carbohydrates. Be aware of:

- High carb veggies, such as squash, mushrooms, garlic, parsnip, onion

- Nightshades, such as peppers, eggplant, tomatoes

- Berries, such as blueberries, raspberries, and blackberries

- Citrus, such as orange juice, lime juice, lemon juice, and zests

- Avoid starchy veggies and larger fruits such as bananas and potatoes

- Here is a list of the best low carb veggies!

- Asparagus

- Avocados

- Bell Peppers

- Broccoli

- Cauliflower

- Green beans

- Kale

- Lettuce

- Mushrooms

- Spinach

- Zucchini

Dairy

Dairy is a very common item on the ketogenic diet, despite popular belief. Even so, you still need to be aware of your consumption of dairy and moderate it. Most of your meals need to be made up of added fats and cooking oils, vegetables, and protein. Organic and raw dairy items are preferred on the ketogenic diet whenever you can purchase them. Dairy that is highly processed has 2-5 times the amount of carbs than raw dairy. Also, you should opt for full-fat dairy items over fat-free and low-fat options, as they have more carbs and tend to be less filling in the long run. Dairy items that are encouraged to eat on the keto diet are:

- Mayo and mayo alternatives
- Hard cheeses, such as swiss, feta, parmesan, aged cheddar, etc.
- Soft cheeses, such as Monterey jack, Colby, blue, brie, mozzarella, etc.
- Spreadable dairy, such as crème fraiche, mascarpone, sour cream, cream cheese, cottage cheese, etc.
- Heavy whipping cream
- Greek yogurt

Dairy is a good way to place additional fats into your meals by making sauces and fattier side dishes, such as creamed spinach. Remember, however, that dairy has protein in it too, so take that into account when pairing dairy items with dishes that are heavy in proteins.

Nuts and Seeds

Nuts and seeds are the best to consume when they are roasted, since this removes any anti-nutrients. Avoid eating peanuts, since they are considered legumes and are not highly permitted when you are undergoing the ketogenic diet.

Raw nuts are a great way to add texture and flavors to your meals. Many people like to eat them as simple snacks, which can be rewarding to your munchies but detrimental to your weight loss goals. Snacking raises insulin levels and leads to slower weight loss in the long run. Nuts are a superb source of fat but remember they still do have a carb count that can add up quickly. They also contain a good amount of protein as well. Nut flours can really make protein consumption add up, so be aware of this. Nuts are also high in omega 6 fatty acids. You will want to opt for the fattier, lower in carb nuts.

- Fatty and low carb nuts should be eaten to supplement fat: Brazil nuts, macadamia nuts, and pecans.

- Fatty and moderate in carb nuts: almonds, hazelnuts, peanuts, pine nuts, and walnuts.

- High in carb nuts should rarely be eaten on the keto: cashews and pistachios.

Water and Beverages

The ketogenic diet is based around a diuretic effect that happens naturally, which makes dehydration a common phenomenon. You know that whole '8 glasses of water per day' rule? You will want to drink that and more. Hydration plays an essential role in our everyday life and how well our bodies function. On the ketogenic diet, it is recommended to drink as close to a gallon of water that you can get per day.

- Water is the obvious healthiest choice and should be considered your staple drink and go-to source for ultimate hydration. Drink it still or sparkling.

- Broth is packed with nutrients and vitamins that your body needs. It also plays a role in kickstarting your energy by replenishing lost electrolytes.

- Coffee helps to improve mental focus and has added weight loss benefits!

- Tea has similar effects as coffee. You should lean towards green or black teas.

- Coconut and almond milks can help you to enjoy your dairy beverages without all the added sugar and carbs.

- Diet sodas should be weaned off and avoided when on any diet, let alone the ketogenic diet. Drinking them can lead to cravings for sugar and result in spikes in insulin.

- Beverage flavorings, such as stevia or sucralose are okay on the keto diet. But a healthier alternative is a squeeze or two of an orange, lime, or lemon.

- Alcohol should be a beverage that you enjoy rarely on the ketogenic diet. Lean towards hard liquors instead of beers and wine, since they have a lower sugar content.

Spices and Cooking

Sauces and seasonings are things that newbie ketogenic dieters struggle with since they are used to using them to add flavor to better enjoy their meals. The easiest thing you can do is to simply avoid the consumption of processed foods. There are handfuls of great low carb condiments and spices, but you want to steer clear of high glycemic sweeteners. Spices also have carbs in them, so ensure where you are adding them really counts.

- Basil
- Cayenne pepper
- Chili power
- Cilantro
- Cinnamon
- Cumin
- Oregano
- Parsley
- Rosemary
- Thyme

Condiments and Sauces

This food group on the ketogenic diet is a pretty grey area. This means if you want to be strict with your diet, you should honestly avoid any sauces and condiments that are pre-made. They tend to have additional sugars that you want to avoid in the first place.

If you choose to create your own gravies and sauces, invest in xanthan gum or guar, which are thickeners that are low in carbs and prevent you from having to eat watery sauces. Yuck. Luckily for you, there is a variety of sauces out there that are low in carbs and high in fat. Flavored syrups that are made with accepted sweeteners. Salad dressings, the fattier, the better:

- unsweetened vinaigrettes, Ranch, and Caesar
- Horseradish
- Worcestershire sauce
- Relish (low or no sugar added)
- Sauerkraut (low or no sugar added)
- Mayonnaise (cage-free and avocado-oil)
- Hot Sauce
- Mustard
- Ketchup (low and no sugar added)

Sweeteners

Steering clear of things that are sweet is your best bet when undergoing the ketogenic diet; this will help to totally curb your sweet tooth cravings, which promotes better keto success. There are some options you can use to make that sweet tooth of yours happy:

- Stevia

- Sucralose
- Erythritol
- Monk fruit
- Various blends of sweeteners (read ingredients!)

Chapter 5:
Shopping List Summary

Ketogenic Vegetables

Artichokes	Cucumbers
Asparagus	Eggplant
Avocados	Spinach
Bean Sprouts	Green bell peppers
Bell peppers (Any color)	Green onions
Bok Choy	Greens
Broccoli	Hot peppers
Brussel Sprouts	Iceberg lettuce
Cabbage	Leeks
Canned artichoke hearts	Mushrooms
Canned asparagus	Napa cabbage
Canned black olives	Okra
Canned green beans	Portabella mushrooms
Canned green olives	Radishes
Canned greens	Romaine lettuce
Canned mushrooms	Snow peas
Canned pickles	Spaghetti squash
Canned sauerkraut	Spinach
Cauliflower	Yellow onions
Celery	Zucchini

Ketogenic Fruits

Apples	Mango

Apricot	Melons
Avocados	Nectarines
Bananas	Olives
Blackberries	Oranges
Blueberries	Papaya
Cherries	Passion fruit
Fresh cranberries	Peaches
Dates	Pears
Figs	Pineapple
Grapefruit	Plums
Guava	Pomegranates
Kiwi	Raspberries
Lemons	Rhubarb
Limes	Strawberries
Tangerines	Tomatoes (all types)

Ketogenic Dairy

Sour cream	Colby cheese
Heavy whipping cream	Cottage cheese
Mayonnaise	Feta cheese
Full fat/full cream Greek yogurt	Goat cheese
Full fat/full cream milk	Monterey Jack cheese
Blue cheese	Mozzarella cheese
Brie cheese	Parmesan cheese
Cheddar cheese	Swiss cheese

Ketogenic Beef

Corned beef	Baby back ribs
Steak	Prime rib
Roast beef	Hamburger
All non-lean cuts of beef	

Ketogenic Pork

Ground pork	Tenderloin
Pork chips	Pork roast
Bacon	Unglazed ham

Ketogenic Poultry

Chicken broth	Chicken eggs
Cornish hens	Whole chicken
Chicken legs, wings, and thighs	Canned chicken (read labels!)
Turkey legs	Ground turkey
Whole turkey	Turkey breast
Duck eggs and meat	Goose eggs and meat
Pheasant eggs and meat	Quail eggs and meat

Ketogenic Seafood

Anchovies	Bass
Canned salmon and tuna	Catfish
Cod	Crab
Flounder	Haddock
Halibut	Herring
Lobster	Orange Roughie
Oysters	Salmon
Sardines	Scallops
Shellfish	Shrimp
Sole	Tilapia
Trout	Tuna fish

Ketogenic Spices

Real bacon bits	All spice
Cajun spice	Capers
Chili powder	Cinnamon

Cream of tartar	Cumin
Dill	Garlic powder
Garlic salt	Horseradish
Hot sauce	Onion powder
Oregano	Paprika
Parsley	Pumpkin spice
Salt	Turmeric
Pepper	

Ketogenic Sauces and Dressings

Soy sauce	Vinegar
Worcestershire sauce	Yellow and brown mustards
Sugar-free ketchup	Sugar-free syrup
Blue cheese	Ranch
Italian	Lemon juice
Lime juice	Low-carb salsa

Ketogenic Liquids

Protein shakes	Unsweetened tea
Coffee with heavy cream	Almond milk
Cashew milk	Coconut milk

Ketogenic Cooking and Baking

Bearnaise sauce	Butter
Bacon fat	Coconut oil
Duck fat	Hollandaise sauce
Mayonnaise	Olive oil
Peanut oil	Sesame oil
Sunflower oil	Coconut flour
Coconut flakes	Almond flour and meal
Flax meal	Flax seeds

| Chia seed | Cocoa powder |

Ketogenic Sweeteners

| Xylitol |
| Stevia drops |
| Erythritol |

Chapter 6:
Greater Keto Success with Clean Eating

Eating 'cleaner' is seen all over social media and on the news as a better way to fuel your body. But many people do not quite understand what qualifies as 'clean eating'. Whether you want to further ensure your success on the Ketogenic Diet or want to step up your diet a notch, clean eating paired with the Ketogenic Diet can yield amazing results! Clean eating is not just a trend; it should be something all of us are doing much more often. Let's learn the basics of clean eating, shall we?

What is 'Clean Eating?'
It is no secret that over the past couple of years, the clean eating trend has gained a lot of traction. But very few people know what it means to "eat clean", how it is beneficial, let alone how to start. I don't blame all these people since society today has made it seem like an impossible feat to incorporate more whole foods into our diet.

Clean eating is a simple concept. Instead of focusing on ingesting more or less of things, such as those diets that focus on fewer calories and more protein, for example, it is about becoming more consciously aware of the pathway that food must take to get from its origin to our plate. Clean eating is centered around eating whole foods, also referred to as 'real foods.' Real foods are those that are not processed, handled, or refined in any way, which makes them closest to their natural form.

What are 'Processed Foods'?

Before we dive deeper into the nutritious world of whole foods, let's take a closer look at what we know to be processed foods. The following is what classifies some consumables as 'processed':

- If there any additions, such as fat, sugar, or salt to add flavor or preservatives to keep food from spoiling, to vitamins.

- Changes in the natural form of the food. For example, taking out the germ and bran from whole grains to make refined bread or mashing apples to make applesauce or stir-frying vegetables.

- Foods that have any lab-created components. Those ingredients you have no clue how to pronounce? Yeah...those ones.

Are All Processed Foods Bad?

Not all processed foods are bad for you to consume. Many times, the processing procedures on what we eat remove bacteria and other toxins so that we can enjoy certain kinds of foods. Processing also includes the act of altering the overall consistency or the taste of things to make it more appealing to our taste buds. Even instant oatmeal, kale smoothies, and pasteurized milk are processed. You just want to avoid eating foods that are overly processed, such as those labeled "ready-to-heat", for instance.

The Dark Side of Ultra-Processed Eats

You can probably only *imagine* the plethora of health issues that are directly linked to the consumption of overly processed foods.

- Foods that combine GMO's or genetically modified organisms have been linked to infertility and cancer.

- Foods that are highly processed are literally stripped of their nutrients that are needed to be healthy.

- Overly processed foods are modified heavily and tend to assist in the overproduction of the pleasure neurotransmitter known as dopamine, which is what causes us to have cravings for junk foods.

Benefits of Clean Eating

Although you are here to counteract your weight and shed some pounds, there are many other perks to a clean diet that stretch way beyond the scale:

- *Healthier gums and teeth.* Since digestion starts in your mouth, getting rid of excess sugary foods and beverages that are loaded with sugar will maintain a healthier environment and cuts down your risk of developing gingivitis and cavities.

- *Shinier hair and stronger nails.* Eating clean makes you consume more vitamins, antioxidants, and omega 3 fatty acids that help the protein in both your nails and hair to be stronger.

- *More energetic.* What you consume for breakfast can often be to blame for wanting to climb under your desk and catch a quick cat-nap midafternoon. If your breakfast lacks protein, your energy is taken away. The first meal of your day should always include whole grains, protein, and healthy fat.

- *More satisfied.* When you consume a well-balanced diet of fats, protein, and whole grain carbs, you are giving your body the energy it needs to sustain itself for hours, which alleviates hunger pangs and cravings.

- *Decreased risk of developing diseases.* Even if you feel great fueling your body with junk right now, you are preparing for a world of hurt later in your life. Foods high in fat, sugar, and sodium have been known to cause diabetes, heart disease, and a few cancers as well.

- *Great mental wellbeing.* When you eat clean, you are more apt to maintain a good physical lifestyle too. Diets that are composed of rich omega 3's have been shown to ward off mood swings and depression. B-vitamins are great to get those feel-good chemicals in the brain moving around and helping you feel your best.

- *More productive.* When you consume foods that are real and whole, you are fueling not only your body but your mind the best you can. This enables you to remain focused.

- *Better quality of sleep.* If you find yourself tossing and turning half the night, you might need to reexamine your bedtime munchies. Skip the candy or leftover takeout and eat foods that are naturally loaded with tryptophan, such as almonds and low-fat milk.

My Favorite Clean Eating Items

As you are aware, eating cleaner is not always the simplest task, especially when unhealthy temptations lurk around every corner at your grocery store and at the office kitchen. You may not be able to eat *every* meal cleanly, but you can take great strides in limiting your intake of processed foods. Here are my personal clean eating favs to get you started on the right track!

- Apples
- Beef
- Carrots
- Chicken
- Corn
- Cream
- Eggs
- Figs
- Garlic
- Ham
- Nuts
- Oranges
- Peaches
- Pineapple
- Soups (made from scratch)
- Soy

- Spinach
- Strawberries
- Turkey
- Yogurt

Beginner's Guide to Shopping Clean

One of the biggest stresses I faced personally, and I know others face as well when it comes to eating cleaner is the dreaded trip to gather supplies at the grocery store.

My first time walking into a store after I made the decision to eat clean was thrilling. I was motivated and ready to take on the world and fuel my body better than ever before. But my motivation started to disappear in the first aisle when I was bombarded by a sea of ingredient lists and labels. By the time I managed to find an appropriate loaf of bread, I was beyond frustrated, and I left the store and didn't even get the bread I took so long to find.

If you have done this before, trust me, I know the feeling of disappointment, coming home and letting your feelings out on that box of slightly stale donuts. But for those that have either attempted to shop clean before or have never done it at all, this portion of the chapter I shall outline an easy to read guide on how to shop clean, the right and frustration-free way. Shopping clean does not have to be a complicated venture. If you have the right approach and mindset, you will be able to conquer that sea of labels and get what you need to pave your path to a healthier you in no time!

Accept that You Will Have to Change

Before you pick any recipes, buy any containers, make a list, or step foot into a store, you need to realize that you are about to make many changes that inevitably come along with choosing to eat cleaner. This means drastically switching up the way you shop. You will also come to find that there is not a substitute for all the things you have always eaten, so it is time to rid your body of these things. Accept that some things are bound to change and be okay with it.

How to Shop Clean

I learned a little trick that all grocery stores do throughout my experience in the beginning process of clean eating. I learned to shop along the perimeters of the store, rather than dwelling in the center. Why? All the items that are clean and fresh are located here. You should avoid the aisles of the store unless you need things such as frozen veggies and chicken or steel cut oats, for instance.

Right when you step over the threshold of the store and grab yourself a cart, head to the perimeter right off the bat. Begin in the produce section and fill your cart with as many fresh items as you can eat in a week's time. Then move to the meat and deli sections, the dairy, etc. The best technique to clean eating is to totally avoid foods that have a label at all. When you think fresh, you can eat cleaner and get in the mindset of packing your cart with real food that has no need for an ingredient list. This will discard over half the frustration right away!

Reading Labels

Expect there to be opportunities where you do end up venturing down an aisle at the store to locate things that might just be slightly processed or not kept along the clean eating perimeters. A big part of cleaner consumption is learning how to properly read labels to ensure you are staying the course.

- *Number of ingredients*: Most recipes have more than five or six ingredients and are still considered clean. In fact, you could have a label of twenty or more clean ingredients, and it is still not processed. So, forego what you have been taught that labels should not have more than five components. This is just not realistic in most cases.

- *Reading labels*: Look at the ingredients singularly first. Are there any that you would purchase separately to cook with in your kitchen at home? Take spaghetti sauce for example. 'Basil, olive oil, garlic and tomatoes' are all clean since you would just have to purchase one of those ingredients to cook with. But if there is something such as 'maltodextrin', which is something hard to pronounce and that you can't buy by itself, put it back.

- *Percentages and grams*: While this section of the label is essential for many people looking for something to buy when it comes to just clean eating, I typically put the ingredient list as a top priority.

Relax and Learn to Move Forward

There are bound to be times that you mistakenly purchase things that are not as clean as you thought. This is not the end of the world and you do not need to take it back. Just remember not to get that item next time. Don't expect perfection right when you are starting the clean eating process. And don't deny your cravings either. Take it one step at a time and pat yourself on the back for trying your best!

Affordable Clean Eating Shopping List

When you are just starting the path down the road to clean eating, it can be hard to know what to get at the store and get the most bang for your buck at the same time. This portion of the chapter is a go-to list I utilize myself often. I hope you find use out of it!

Grains

- Whole grain bread

- Ezekiel brand bread

- Whole wheat crackers

- Whole wheat tortillas, preferably ones that are made with water, lime, and/or corn.

Dairy and Non-Dairy

- Milk: the best would be raw milk with other options including organic and full-fat milk.

- Cottage cheese: full fat is the best but low-fat can be used.

- Yogurt: Greek yogurt is the best with plain yogurt as another great option

- Cheese: real grated parmesan cheese (cheeses are eaten on clean eating diets in moderation since they are so high in fat).

- Non-dairy: unsweetened almond milk, unsweetened rice milk, untweeted soymilk, and untweeted coconut milk.

Poultry
- Eggs

- Chicken and turkey (boneless and skinless poultry breasts will become your best friends on your clean eating venture).

- Beef: opt for grass-fed so don't be afraid to try buffalo, bison, and venison as well!

- Other meats: pork, duck, venison, fish (most fish are considered clean eating).

Produce
This is the section that you cart should be overflowing with by the end of your shopping trip. My rule of thumb is to stick to organics when it comes to items that have thin skins, such as berries and peaches. Then, you can purchase regular items with thicker skins, such as oranges and bananas.

Fruits
- Star fruit

- Kiwi

- Cherries
- Berries
- Avocados
- Bananas
- Grapefruits
- Oranges
- Apples
- Any other enjoyable fresh fruit

Vegetables
- Onions
- Sweet potatoes
- Tomatoes
- Green beans
- Okra
- Collard greens
- Chard
- Kale
- Squash

- Eggplant
- Zucchini
- Bell peppers
- Broccoli
- Spinach
- Celery
- Carrots

The Aisles

- Tea: Go green!
- Coffee
- Oatmeal: Don't get flavored oatmeal. Stick with steel cut or traditionally rolled.
- Canned items: Ensure there is no added sugar and watch the content of sodium
- Dry legumes and beans
- Brown rice
- Whole wheat or whole grain brown rice and pasta
- Other whole grains, like barley, etc.
- Nuts and seeds

- Condiments, spices, and sweeteners

- Ketchup: it's almost impossible to find clean ketchup to buy in stores. But you *can easily make your own at home.*

- Mustard: Mustard without loaded extra sugars is hard to locate. I personally like the OrganicVille brand because it has a good taste without all the additional sugar. If you cannot find it, opt for Dijon and other mustard varieties.

- Honey: The healthiest version of honey you can consume is Manuka honey

- Pure maple syrup

- Molasses

- Spices: Most herbs can be bought in bulk and you can freeze them for later use!

Flours
- Almond flour

- Coconut flour

- White whole wheat flour

- Whole wheat flour

- Whole wheat pastry flour

Clean Superfoods You Can Get for $1 or Less

Superfoods have become one of my absolute favorite parts of my clean eating journey. They are not only all the rage, but they can be made in a tremendous variety of ways and plus, they are super cheap! Talk about doubly super foods!

- *Lentils* have 8 grams of fiber per half a cup and 9 grams of protein, which makes them excellent for heart health. They even have an edge over bean consumption, especially in terms of preparation. They take just 15 to 30 minutes and do not require to be soaked beforehand. One cup of lentils is just 20 cents.

- *Oats* are the best soluble fiber you can consume, with 3 grams per serving. When you increase your consumption of this type of fiber by 5 to 10 grams per day, you can drop your bad cholesterol by 5 percent. Quick cook oats are just as great as steel cut ones, just ensure you avoid oatmeal packets because they are packed with additional sugars. 1/3 of a cup of oats is just 10 cents.

- *Kale* is one of the most renowned of the superfoods with a cup holding ten times the value of vitamin K which is great for your bone health. It also includes three times the value of vitamin A, which assists in vision health. One cup of kale costs only 77 cents.

- *Almonds* hold 37 percent of the daily value of vitamin E in just a one ounce serving. This is one of the nutrients that so many people never consume enough of. They help give your body folate, fiber, and calcium as well. An ounce of almonds, which is about 23 nuts, costs 63 cents.

- *Tea* is not only super-healthy for you but is very budget-friendly too. Green tea especially is loaded with antioxidants which help to boost your immune system and promote a healthy heart. There have been studies that found that drinking just twelve ounces of green or black tea per day were less likely to have a heart attack than those that never consumed tea. One tea bag is just a dime.

- *Oranges* provide you with your daily value of vitamin C and give you 3 grams of fiber. It satisfies your stomach with just 70 calories. Also, that bright orange color means that they boost beta-carotene, which promotes better vision. An orange is just 34 cents.

- *Tuna* is loaded with omega-3s. Consuming it just two times per week can help you to lower cholesterol levels. A 3 ounce can of tuna costs around 48 to 77 cents.

- *Peanut butter* is not only yummy on the taste buds but is highly versatile. It improves cholesterol and lowers the chance of developing heart disease. It is loaded with zinc, vitamin E, and healthy fats. Opt for natural peanut butter so you can cut out unnecessary oils and sugars. Two tablespoons of natural peanut butter are around 21 cents.

- *Eggs* are packed with essential nutrients in such an inexpensive package. The whites alone hold 4 grams of protein and the yolks are packed with vitamin D, which helps in decreasing macular degeneration that is age-related. For only 80 calories, who wouldn't eat eggs? And one egg is only 17 cents.

- *Apples* hold tangible heart-related benefits and have been shown to improve overall health for those that consume two apples per day. One apple is around 28 cents.

- *Carrots* give your body a nice dose of beta-carotene and give you four times the amount of vitamin A, which contributes to bone health and immune functioning. A cup of carrots is just 23 cents.

- *Cabbage*, just like kale, is rich in vitamins K and C and provides consumers with tons of fiber. At only around 22 calories per serving and 25 cents per cup, regular and red cabbage is a must to add to your clean eating list.

Chapter 7:
Meal Prepping on the Keto Diet

There are many people that aspire to live a healthier lifestyle but have no idea where to start or have no time to spare. Eating healthy is one thing but following through with your health and fitness goals and staying consistent is challenging.

When you have your hands full navigating life, cooking all our own meals can feel impossible and the temptations of hitting up a fast food joint seem like an easier option. If you are ready to reach your fitness goals, stop spending extraordinary amounts of money on junk food, then your new best friend is meal prepping!

What is Meal Prepping?
Meal prepping is planning, preparing, and packaging snacks and meals for the upcoming week with the idea of portion control and clean eating in mind. There is no right or wrong way to meal prep, which makes it a great dieting alternative for busy bees to personalize to fit into their daily schedule. The goal of meal prepping is to save substantial time slaving away in the kitchen while having access to healthier meal options throughout the week. You simply dedicate time for planning your meals and cooking their components. Besides that, you will become *amazed* at the difference meal prepping will make in your day to day life!

Reasons Why You Should Be Meal Prepping

- Effective weight loss: When you plan your meals in advance, you will know what you are putting into your body. A meal prep routine lets you control how many calories you consume, which is essential for weight loss.

- Saves money: Despite popular belief, eating healthy doesn't have to be pricey. Purchasing things in bulk and taking advantage of your freezer is key. You know exactly what to buy instead of purchasing ingredients you don't need. Plus, with meals already made, you will save a ton of money on fast food meals.

- Shopping is simpler: Once you plan your week's meals, grocery shopping will be a breeze since you will have a list to stick to instead of wandering around the store.

- Learn portion control: Meal prep teaches you how to balance what you put inside your body. When you pack your meals in containers, it keeps you from reaching for more food that you don't need. This is essential if you want to lose weight; meal prepping allows you to control the nutrients and calories you eat.

-

- Less waste: Meal prepping lets you utilize all your ingredients for the week before they go bad! This is a much better alternative then trashing expensive produce before you have a chance to eat it.

- Saves time: While you will need to set time aside to prepare your meals, you will end up saving time in the long run. Think about it; how much time do you spend with the fridge open? How much time do you waste deciding of what to eat just to become a victim of tempting convenience foods?

With meal prep, meals are prepared ahead of time, requiring you to remove from the fridge and nuke them in the microwave. Easy!

- Investment in your health: When you can pick what you are going to stuff your face ahead of time, you have ample time to make much healthier decisions. The benefits of eating cleaner are endless! Good nutrition is everything, especially if you are looking to fit into that bikini for the summer!

- Strengthens willpower: Once you become accustomed to eating healthier, you will find that you no longer crave sugar and carbs. When you have a consistent routine of eating better, you will be able to turn down unhealthy food choices much easier.

- Reduces stress: Stress directly impacts your immune system, which can cause you to experience digestive issues, lack of quality sleep, and many more negative side effects. Coming home from work and having a meal ready to eat takes away that everyday stress!

- Adds variety to your diet: Once you get the hang of meal prepping, you will feel more confident to try new recipes with new ingredients. Your taste buds will receive a variety of flavor daily.

Fundamentals of Meal Prep

Pantry Tips: There are many other items besides fruits, veggies, and canned goods that can reside happily in a pantry. These tips pertain to foods in storage that don't need to be frozen or refrigerated:

- To lengthen the time of prepper foods, store them in plastic or glass meal prep containers.

- Most canned foods that are low in acids, such as vegetables, crab meat, and tuna can last 2 to 5 years. Ensure you check the date.

- Canned foods that are high in acid, like tomato-based items, pineapple, and grapefruit have a shelf life of 12 to 18 months.

- Conditions of storage areas should be cool, dark, and dry with temps that range from 50 to 70 degrees. Warm climates make food deteriorate faster, so keep items away from hot pipes, dishwasher, and oven.

Fridge Tips
- Stay alert for spoiled food. If anything looks or smells off, it should be thrown out. Yes, mold can happen in the fridge too.

- Keep prepped meals covered and in plastic or glass containers, wrapped in foil or plastic wrap.

- Pay attention to expiration dates

- Be vigilant of the 2-hour rule of refrigeration, meaning not leaving items that require to be chilled out for more than 2 hours, such as dairy, seafood, eggs, meat, chicken, etc.

- Set the temp in your fridge to 40 degrees or lower

Freezer Tips: I want to nicely remind you that freezing meals does not kill bacteria, but it can stop it from growing. Most frozen foods can last for a long time, but the color, flavor, and tenderness of frozen items can be affected the longer they are frozen.

- Thaw food in your fridge before prepping

- Don't fear freezer burn; it's a quality of food issue, not a food safety problem

- Label all packages you freeze with the date, what food is in it, and any other identifying information that will help your meal prep efforts, such as what it weighs or how many servings are in the container

- Ensure that you properly wrap food you wish to freeze; utilize airtight storage contains, and use bags, plastic wrap, and foil that is freezer-grade

- Set the temp of your freezer to 0 degrees or below

Freezer vs. Fridge: Freeze your meals if you don't plan to consume then in 3 to 4 days after you prepare them. Remember that prepping frozen meals takes a bit more preparation time than refrigerated meals.

- Thaw out meals for a few hours or overnight before heating and consuming.

- Frozen meals last substantially longer than refrigerated meals, some being able to be frozen up to one year.

Keep in mind not all edibles are freezer friendly, foods such as fruits high in water content, lettuce, uncooked batters, eggs, cooked pasta, soft cheeses, and cultured dairy are not suitable.

Refrigerated meals are capable of being tasty, fresh, and convenient for a few days. After prepping, you just must nuke the meals in the microwave. After several days of living in the fridge, however, meals can lose their freshness, taste, and moisture. This is because dry air circulating takes the moisture out of food.

Refrigerate Meals You Plan to Eat in 3 to 4 Days

Meal prepping is much more than spending Sunday afternoons prepping various meals to consume throughout the week and stuffing them in containers to tote around. There are many ways people go wrong when they make the great decision to venture down the path of prepping meals. This chapter is full of things to keep you in mind to get you started as well as great tips and tricks to make the most out of prepping!

Getting Started

Here are some great aspects to keep in mind when beginning your journey into the world of meal prepping.

- *Choose a Cooler Bag.* There are many types of cooler bags in every shape, size, and color. I recommend you investigate brands such as Fitmark, Six Pack Fitness, and Isolator Fitness. While some offer not only the bag but containers and ice packs too, you can easily purchase all these items separately as well.

- *Choose Containers*: You will want to investigate containers that are microwave and freezer safe that are also BPA free. Finding just the right containers seems to be a common issue for those starting to meal prep. The company Isolater Fitness offers many shapes and sizes of containers to choose from.

- Sizes of containers make a big impact. For an older gentleman, they may eat three 16-ounce containers each day before a specific time. You may need less or more than this.

Planning Out Your First Meals

Many individuals consume their prepped meals outside of the comfort of their own homes, which means you need to keep these factors in mind when planning your first days of prepping:

- *Stay away from soups.* These liquid-based foods are a hassle which makes you more susceptible to making a mess and wearing more than you eat.

- *Find meals that reheat well.* Plan out meals that you can pop in the toaster oven or microwave. Things with sauces and dressings typically do poorly, as well as many fish items.

- *Find meals that don't need a knife.* Meals that need a lot of time to cut can be a hassle as well, especially if you are eating it in your lap, etc. If you have pork chops or chicken breasts of anything similar, make sure to cut them up into bite-sized pieces before putting in a container.

Meal Prep Step-by-Step

When it comes to beginning your journey into meal prep, you need to remember not to let yourself become overwhelmed. I know I managed to bog myself down as a newbie with all the details that people put out there, instead of just focusing on the basics. When you get the basics down, then perhaps you can start to think more about the nitty-gritty.

My number one recommendation when first starting out prepping is to incorporate as few things at once time. For instance, don't attempt to prep meals with all new, healthy recipes. You should begin by prepping recipes you already know and probably like. This will help you to feel comfortable. Once you get the hang of prepping meals you are familiar with, then you can venture more into the unknown world of healthy recipes galore.

There are many people that get on those health kicks and then quickly lose their gusto since there are just too many things happening all at once. Change, no matter what size, is a big deal. If you try to make too many at once, you are likely to throw in the towel. For instance, start with eating only salad for lunch, making sure you make the gym a priority, etc. during the first week and work your way up. You are setting yourself up for better success this way. Baby steps are key when implementing meal prepping techniques into your life. This portion of the chapter will cover a step-by-step guide to meal prepping.

Step One: Start Out Small

As you have learned, prepping meals is a tried and true way to fuel your body in a healthier fashion. It creates a barrier against temptation and gives you the advantage to make healthy choices in the first place. As a beginner, you are not going to be accustomed to cooking in batches, so I would start just prepping one to two days' worth of meals to begin with.

Starting small gives you time to get used to all the steps it takes to prep, from chopping, cooking, cleaning and more. If you try to do too much at the beginning, you will lose momentum due to being overwhelmed. Starting small also gives you the opportunity to try a few newer recipes to see how much you like them and to see if you really want to devour them. You don't want to make a bunch of food and then waste it.

Step Two: Kitchen Essentials
Thankfully, you don't need a bunch of fancy equipment in your kitchen to make healthy meals right at home. Here are the basics tools you will need and find mighty helpful as your meal prep:

- Baking sheet
- Blender or food processor
- Chef's knife
- Cutting board
- Instant pot or slow cooker
- Mason jars
- Meal prep containers
- Measuring spoons and cups
- Mixing bowls
- Sauté pan
- Small saucepan
- Spatula

Step Three: Choose a Day

First things first, pick out a day that you will dedicate yourself to preparing meals. Sunday is typically the best for most people since they are usually off work and have more time to do it. Plus, meals are fresher for the week ahead. And if you have kids, they are off from school so enlist their tiny hands to help!

For me personally, I choose two days a week, Sunday and Wednesday. This allows me to split up the prepping for the week into two days. When you first start out, do not make the mistake I did by attempting to prepare the meals for the whole week. Instead, I recommend starting off by making three meals at a time. I am a very visual person, so I began keeping a calendar to literally map out my meals. I have a physical calendar in my kitchen dedicated to meal prepping. IF you find that a calendar on your mobile device works better, then, do what works best for you!

Step Four: Choose Meals

Now it is time to make the choice of which meals to make first: Breakfast, Lunch or, Dinner? If you are prepping for an entire family, then you should stick to putting most of your effort into dinner prep. If you are single or cooking just for two, then I would recommend making breakfast and lunch meals first. The choice is yours at the end of the day, but make sure to put at least some thought into it before you get your hands dirty.

Once you decided what course to prepare, now you can pick which recipes! Even though you can cook the same recipes for all three meals, you may not want to. When picking out recipes to make, it is important to think about the overall balance of that meal. Are you trying to maintain specific goals related to macronutrients like carbs, fats, and proteins? Then these should play a factor in those recipes. I find it helpful to know how each of those nutrients converts into calories in picking out meals to make:

- 1 gram of protein is equivalent to 4 calories

- 1 gram of carbohydrates is equivalent to 4 calories

- 1 gram of fat is equivalent to 9 calories

Once you have a list of recipes, obviously you need to ensure you have all the components to create them! Check your pantry and fridge first and make a list of the things you need so you don't stray to the dark side at the grocery store. I find it handy to use a kitchen scale so that you can disperse each portion of your meals evenly. Which ties into step five…

Step Five: Ensure You Have Correct Containers

I cannot stress to you enough the importance of having the proper containers when it comes to meal prepping. In fact, quality storage containers are the foundation to prepping because how you store meals can either make or break all that effort. You don't want to just dump meals into Tupperware bowls, for this defeats the purpose of prepping. If you throw it all into one container, foods get mixed and become a big pile of nasty goop. So, what makes a good container?

- Airtight

- BPA free (safe and microwaveable)

- Clear

- Divided sections

- Freezer and dishwasher safe
- Reusable
- Same size
- Stackable

For me personally, I found that the square and/or rectangle 24-ounce containers are awesome to pack lunches and the ½ - 1 cup containers are great for snacks. I often utilize snack-size zip baggies to store snack combos, since they guys are made for portion control.

Step Six: In the Kitchen

Like we have mentioned before, you need to start off your meal prep journey with beginning to prep just a couple to a few meals at a time. You can gradually make more meals in one sitting as time goes on and you become more comfortable with the meal prep process. You want to find your groove first!

Plan to set aside one to two days out of your week to cook batches of food. For instance, I like to cook on Sundays mainly so that I can prepare most of the week ahead. I also occasionally cook Wednesdays, making parts of meals that will last three to four days and cooking again when I am out.

Cook all your protein you plan to use at the same time. For instance, while chicken breasts are cooking away in the oven, make a batch of turkey burgers. If you are cooking five chicken breasts at once, season each with different spices so that your taste buds do not become bored.

If you are a vegetarian, then cook up batches of lentils or beans while baking firm tofu, for example.

You will learn to see the world of vegetables in a different light. Veggies can be raw, roasted, stir-fired, or steamed. I suggest always trying to cut up your vegetables into like-size chunks so that everything gets completely cooked at the right time. Roasted veggies are my personal favorite! It brings out all that sweetness that is naturally in them. Make sure to add dried or fresh herbs and coconut or olive oil to create a delicious flavor.

Grains can be cooked all at once for the entire week. A pot of amaranth, brown rice, or quinoa will last you five days. Bake some spaghetti squash, butternut squash, or sweet potatoes at the same time you are cooking grains.

If you have a slow cooker or instant pot in your arsenal of kitchen appliances, then you are already ahead of the game. You can dump everything in either of these or let the machine do all the hard work for you. The instant pot is also my favorite way to make homemade oatmeal!

Breakfast, as we all know, is a crucial meal to start out the day since it starts up your metabolism and gives both your mind and body the fuel it needs to work hard. Breakfast also acts as a barrier against those terrible cravings that we all tend to have later in the day.

Some of my favorite breakfast items are high-protein pancakes, overnight oats, high-protein muffins, and mini-frittatas. You can whip up a big batch of each and freeze the portions you do not cook right away.

Once you become comfortable cooking meal prep eats, you will learn about the awesomeness of preparing staples ahead of time. Staples can be anything from yams, lentils, oats, rice, etc. These items typically take the longest to make. For instance, when I make rice, I make enough for the meal that day, chill a portion and then freeze the rest to utilize for later recipes.

Chapter 8:
Meal Prep Basics Recap

Create A Meal Plan
Set time aside each week to think about the meals you want to prepare for yourself. Create a meal plan and know what ingredients you have already and which ones you need to go out and purchase. Stick to staple-like items when planning your meals.

- Fruits

- Healthy fats, such as peanuts, almonds, avocado, extra virgin olive oil

- Carbs, such as black, red, or brown rice, sweet potatoes, and wheat bread

- Veggies, such as radishes, snow peas, zucchini, cabbage, bell pepper, cucumber, asparagus, carrots, spinach, green beans, broccoli, etc.

- Proteins, such as yogurt, almond milk, beef, turkey, fish, chicken, eggs

- Avoid soup-like dishes, for these are difficult to store in containers without causing spills.

- Pick a day to prep meals for the week.

- Pick the proper container to store prepped meals in to maintain quality and freshness. Ensure you pick what is best for you regarding portion control.

- Cook all your meat choices. I would suggest getting yourself a nice meat thermometer to ensure your meat is not overdone or undercooked. Trust me, overcooked meat is not fun to heat up and reheat later.

- Use safe food handling procedures when meal prepping. This will help to avoid diseases that are food-borne. You never want to play a part in putting your health in jeopardy.

How to Build a Healthy Meal

As I started my journey into creating better eating habits for myself, I learned that I was viewing food in totally the wrong way. I viewed it as entertainment rather than nourishment. I realize that each meal you eat acts as a building block when it comes to building your overall eating style. To create the best meals to fuel your body, ensure that you are getting all the food groups throughout each day. This means incorporating protein, dairy, grain, vegetables, and fruits and limiting your intake of sodium, saturated fats, and excess sugars.

- Half of your plate should contain fruits and vegetable (opt for fruits that are orange and red or veggies that are dark green).

- Ensure that half of the grains you consume are whole grains ("100-percent whole grains" or "100-percent whole wheat").

- Complete meals with one cup of low-fat or fat-free milk. If you are not a milk fan, try soymilk or include low-fat yogurt as a snack.

- Include lean proteins like tofu, beans, nuts, eggs, turkey, chicken, pork, or lean beef. Try to add seafood as a protein here and there as well.

- Discard items that are heavy in fats and lean towards healthier alternatives.

- Try new foods! Keep your meal prep diet interesting and your taste buds on point by trying recipes and other items that you have never even thought to eat before, such as sardines, kale, quinoa, lentils, and mango.

- Learn to satisfy your sweet tooth in healthier ways by using fruit, such as baked apples. Yum

Remember that everything you consume matters and adds up. Therefore, it is so important to have the right mix of food throughout the day to ensure your overall health is in check.

Must-Haves for Meal Prepping

Meal prepping becomes a heck of a lot simpler when you have the right tools to use in your kitchen. There are links you can click on for each of my favorites that I have personally used or am using currently to ensure my meal prepping goes smoothly. (No, I am not an affiliate for any of these products.)

- Quality meal prep containers that will last.

- Stackable salad containers that can be used for just about anything and can easily be stored in your fridge, freezer, or lunch box.

- Portion control containers to measure out snacks and portions of meals.

- Mason jars for salads, overnight oats, and much more.

- A scale that can be easily read to ensure proper portion control.

- Combination appliances, such as a slow cooker, rice cooker, and steamer all in one.

- A nice set of Pyrex containers to make it easier to store larger batches of food for the week.

- If you love hard-boiled eggs as much as I do, then you will need one of the Dash Go machines that is capable of hard-boiling eggs in just 10 minutes!

- If you are a busy body like I am, then you need to have a quality cooler bag that allows you to tote around multiple meals per day.

- If you are a smoothie-fanatic like yours truly, I came across this personal blender that has drastically changed the way I enjoy smoothies.

Avoiding Common Meal Prep Mistakes

The way you approach meal prepping will make a world of difference when it comes to successfully implementing it into your everyday life. There are many tips out there regarding choosing recipes, shopping, and bringing it all together to create a week's worth of delicious eats. However, you need to be aware of the things that could potentially go wrong and be knowledgeable of solutions to avoid meal prep pitfalls.

Mistake 1: Not Giving Yourself Enough Time to Plan

Meal planning takes time and cannot happen in an hour. When you plan, shop, and prep as soon as you can, you are not giving yourself an enough time to process everything, which can make it more of a stressful experience than it must be.

Solution: Allow yourself ample time to plan meals, especially as a beginner. Set aside 2 to 3 hours per week. Take advantage of the weekend to spread out planning, shopping, and prepping of meals. This will allow prepping to feel like a sustainable task that you can do for months to come.

Mistake 2: Not Choosing the Best Recipes for Your Personal Needs

To ensure that meal prepping works the best for you and your lifestyle, you need to understand the importance of what your body needs from the recipes you choose. If you pick a bunch of recipes that don't come close to the criteria, you will be hungry and unsatisfied.

Solution: Choose recipes based on the meals you need. While this seems obvious, many people overlook this. Create a list of what you want recipes to do for you.

- Need recipes to be 30 minutes or less?
- Are you a vegetarian?
- What ingredients do you have that need to be used?

Mistake 3: Being Unrealistic and too Ambitious

Meal planning should be viewed as a marathon, not a sprint to the finish. You will feel super inspired at the start of your meal prep journey, but once you start to get into the depths of planning, you can become easily overwhelmed.

You need to ensure your prep schedule matches your regular schedule, so you can sustain it.

Solution: Begin by creating defined goals and assessing your daily routine and schedule; this will help you to find what is realistic for you. Start small and start prepping 2 to 3 nights per week. This will give you the opportunity to figure out what works and what doesn't and allows you to tweak it to your liking.

Mistake 4: Not Stocking the Pantry

Meal planners that have experience know how essential it is to always have meal basics on hand. If you fail to keep a good supply of staple items, you will miss all the benefits of meal planning and will likely become susceptible to temptation.

Solution: Stock your pantry with all the basics that you can use time and time again in a variety of recipes.

- Canned goods
- White wine vinegar
- Pepper, salt, and other spices
- Canned tomatoes
- Natural sweeteners (agave, maple, honey)
- Coconut milk
- Olive oil

- Stock

- Etc.

Even on the days you feel like you have nothing to consume, those basic components can help you create a yummy frittata, a delicious three-ingredient entre, or a one-pot wonder.

Mistake 5: Not Searching for Items that Need to be Used Up
Before you head to the store, take inventory of ingredients you already have in your kitchen and make use of leftover components you have. It's a simple step that helps you to prevent waste and saves you money.

Solution: Before choosing recipes and making a grocery list, look in your cupboards, pantry, and fridge for food that needs to be used first. Turn those greens into a tasty side before going bad or thaw that pack of chicken to create a delicious main course.

Mistake 6: Not Jotting Down Recipes
Meal prepping is all about being organized is you want to be successful. If you fail to save or write down recipes you have enjoyed, you will fall off track and become overwhelmed.

Solution: Stay organized by keeping track of recipes that you have enjoyed and new ones you want to try out. It doesn't have to be fancy; could be a scrap piece of paper or on a white board in your kitchen.

Mistake 7: Not Taking Inventory Before Shopping

Once you have picked your recipes for the week, you need to see what items you already have in your pantry. This is a closely tied mistake to not seeing the ingredients that need to be used before going bad.

Solution: Before heading to the store, double check your recipe and the list of ingredients. Check your kitchen to ensure you don't have any of the components already, so you prevent overbuying.

Mistake 8: Skipping Simple Meal Prep

Meal prepping is obviously an essential part of meal prep; this gives your future self a giant hand. If you skip it, you are hurting yourself and leaves more work to do on the weekends.

Solution: Set aside 30 minutes to an hour of prep each evening. This will make weekend meal prep a heck of a lot more efficient.

Mistake 9: Trying New Recipes Each Day

I highly encourage you to try new recipes, but it's also important to go about eating a new variety of foods in a strategic way. When you fill up the whole week with brand new recipes, it can become very overwhelming and hard to sustain over a long period of time.

Solution: Don't throw new recipes to the side but build your meal plan around recipes you know and then add 1 or 2 new recipes per week. This will help your taste buds from becoming bored and will also strengthen your recipe collection.

Mistake 10: Failing to Have a Backup Plan

Even the most experienced meal preppers are bound to get stuck at work or have evenings where they are not feeling like consuming the dinner they planned out. Having a plan B is essential to staying the course.

Solution: Have a good backup plan and have recipes in your back pocket that you know how to make. These will be very simple and can be made quickly, such as an omelet.

Food Storage and Reheating Tips

When you are prepping meals for the week ahead, the max you should prepare is 5 days at a time. This allows you to keep 3 days of meals in the fridge by putting the rest in the freezer. The temperatures that you keep your freezer and fridge are important, especially depending on the type of containers you are using to ensure your meals remain fresh.

- The fridge should be 40 degrees F or below

- The freezer should be 0 degrees F or below

- Preparing hot meals? Let them cool before storing and chilling them.

Glass containers are the best to use when storing in the fridge since you can view the contents of the container and can be microwaved. If you are using plastic containers, ensure they are BPA free. Planning to freeze meals, ensure the containers you are using are airtight, so your meals do not become freezer burnt. Confused on suggested food storage times?

When you plan to defrost meals, take them out the night before the day you plan to consume them. This may take a bit longer, but it is worth it, trust me. If you are faced with having to microwave your meals to defrost, be careful.

Many times, your food will heat quickly and can cause present bacteria to spread. Some portions of your meal will likely be ice cold while other parts are scorching hot.

Smoothie Tips

Put smoothie ingredients for each smoothie into containers or sealable baggies and ensure you only prep just 4 days ahead. Then, all you must do is dump those contents into a blender and push go! Create smoothie ice cubes by blending leftover fruits and veggies and pouring them into ice molds. You can add these to smoothies later instead of using ice that waters down smoothies.

Prep Multitasking in the Kitchen

Learn to cook multiple items all at once. You can bake proteins and roast veggies all in the oven at one time. Do your best to use hearty vegetables that you can roast in just half an hour. This will greatly lessen your time spent in the kitchen. My favorite roasted veggie recipe:

- *Ensure your oven is preheated to 420 degrees.*
- *Chop up veggies. I love putting broccoli, carrots, red potatoes, purple fingerling potatoes, and sweet potatoes.*
- *Combine 2 to 3 tbsp. of olive oil, 1 tsp. oregano, a squeeze of lemon juice, 1 ½ tsp. garlic powder, and 2 sprigs of rosemary together.*
- *Pour the oil mixture over veggies and mix well to ensure even coating.*

- *Pour coated veggies onto a baking sheet and sprinkle with sea salt and pepper.*
- *Bake 30 minutes.*

Get the Most Out of Your Chicken

Since chicken is the most popular form for most meat-lovers on a clean eating diet, here are some tips to get the most out of your favorite meat source:

- Cook different seasoned portions of chicken to ensure variety in your diet and to make sure your taste buds never get bored.
- My favorite trick I learned is to use foil and create 3 portions on a baking sheet and cook three differently seasoned chicken portions all at one time!
- When you are getting yourself used to practicing portion control, make kabobs so that you are more apt to meet the macronutrient requirements
- Wrap chicken over vegetables so that you are consuming veggies and protein at one time.

Get the Most Out of Your Quinoa

Quinoa has become a major staple for me in my clean eating journey personally, as I am sure it has for many others. There are tons of ways to make quinoa tasty and you can do so by just incorporating it with a few ingredients! To make breakfast quinoa:

- Mix with dried berries, a tablespoon of cinnamon, pumpkin seeds, walnuts, etc.

- Scoop out just a cup each morning and heat in microwave for 60 seconds.

- Pour ½ a cup of coconut or almond milk over your quinoa. So much tastier than carb-filled cereals.

For Mediterranean-inspired quinoa for lunch or dinner just add cilantro, pepper, sea salt, cumin, lemon juice, feta cheese, tomatoes, olives, and cucumber and mix well. YUM!

Slow Cooking Tips

Utilizing a slow cooker is a superb way to make quality meals in bulk ahead of time. They are extremely easy to clean and operate as well. This chapter is full of great tips to keep in mind as you dust off your good ole slow cooker and start creating delectable ketogenic slow cooker recipes!

If you don't have a cooker that is programmable, there are plug-in attachments that you can buy. There are several that allow you to set a temperature and cook time. Add dairy products towards the end of cooking: If you heat dairy products for a long time within a cooker, this can make them curdle.

Add pasta, veggies and cooked beans towards the end of cooking too: while sauces have the potential to cook low and slow for a while, to keep pasta al dente you will want to add these types of ingredients in towards the end. You do not want veggies and beans to turn to mush during the process of cooking.

Stews, chilies, and recipes that don't require you to constantly stir them are good to cook overnight: These sorts of recipes will have bigger, bolder taste since they have a chance to sit and merry.

Give hot foods time to cool: You do not want to store extremely hot foods in plastic. This may cause containers to melt. You can make cooling faster by putting the liner in an ice bath if you so choose.

Don't open the lid until you must: If the recipe calls for you to stir the contents or add additional ingredients, these are the only times you should be opening the lid. Many times, slow cookers can take half an hour to regain the temperature in which you have it set.

Don't just use cooker for meat: There are a large variety of snacks, cocktails and easy to make desserts that you can make in the means of a slow cooker.

- Learn to convert oven recipes to make in the slow cooker.
- Fattier cuts of meat are the best to slow cook.
- Brown meats on the stove to build flavor.
- Cook overnight instead of during the day to avoid overcooking.
- Maximize meal planning by incorporating freezer meals into slow cooker arsenal.

Clean up fast by utilizing slow cooker liners: You will no longer have to soak your slow cooker liner in the sink for hours after cooking. Use one of these convenient liners by simply throwing it away after cooking.

- Fill cooker with water till it reaches the ring you wish to remove.

- Pour 1 cup of white vinegar into a 6 quart and ½ cup into a 3 quart.

- Pour in 1 cup of baking soda for a 6 quart and ½ cup for a 3 quart. Make sure to only add one spoonful of soda at a time.

- Turn slow cooker on to low and set for 4 hours.

- Once finished, shut off cooker. Remove lid and allow to cool.

- Empty into the sink and clean out with soapy hot water.

Chapter 9:
The Principles of the Ketogenic Reset Diet

Even though many people have had success when they underwent the Ketogenic Diet, it can be very difficult to ditch your beloved carbs and sweets. Pair that with the possibility of experiencing the keto flu and that can be enough to break the toughest people.

Introducing the Keto Reset Diet
Thankfully, there is a diet that can now prepare you for the big switch to the Ketogenic Diet, known as the Keto Reset Diet. Created by Mark Sisson, who is the founds of the *Primal Kitchen*, it helps to change the method in which your body prefers to fuel itself, which is essentially what the keto diet is in the first place. The biggest difference is that the reset diet gets you into ketosis and used to the transition at a slower pace.

The Keto Reset Diet is a guide that leads people step-by-step into ketosis; essentially, it helps to "dumb down" the entire process and helps those to execute it properly. This is great since the keto diet itself is not the easiest diet to take on. This reset diet allows those that do it to ease into the ketogenic diet with a 21-day transition period that cuts carb consumption so that the transition to the real ketogenic diet doesn't take so much out on your body. The Keto Reset Diet is great for beginners!

For those three weeks that you are on the reset diet, you will be asked to eliminate refined grains and breads, starchy veggies, and other simple sugars. This will help your body to become better at burning fat and it encourages you to go for longer periods without feeling hunger pains as you increase your energy at the same time. When your body begins to become more adapted to the increase in fat consumption, you are then ready to move to the full-blown ketogenic diet. Once you complete that 21 days of the reset diet, the goal is to be able to switch to the full ketogenic diet mode, where you will be expected to cut back more on carbs and eliminate the starchy veggies. With this slow transition, you will likely forego experiencing the keto flu altogether, or at the very least lessen its negative symptoms.

Chapter 10:
The Keto Diet and Intermittent Fasting

Every day you hop onto social media, it is hard to miss the plethora of articles that talk about the benefits of the ketogenic diet and how you can lose weight while doubling your energy. But if you really want to kick that excess weight to the curb and boost those fat-burning results, then pairing your ketogenic diet with the power of intermittent fasting can help you accelerate your results as well as stimulate other performance-boosting benefits.

What is Intermittent Fasting?

Intermittent fasting is essentially a method to supplement your diet and resolves around the timing of when you consume food. On any diet, let alone the keto, your amount of success is dictated by how much fat and protein you eat, when you eat, how often, and how much you consume. All these factors impact the way your body functions. Whether you have had your results on the keto plateau, or you are just researching the best practices to implement for success on the ketogenic diet, then intermittent fasting is a great option. Fasting is not a requirement to lose weight on this diet. Remember that restricting yourself in unrealistic ways is very pointless; it is not worth going through being unhappy to lose weight. You will just gain it back over time.

The Approach of Intermittent Fasting

The two most important words you need to understand in intermittent fasting are fasting and feeding.

- Your body is in a state of feeding when you are consuming food.

- Your body is in a state of fasting when you are in-between meals.

- The different types of approaches to intermittent fasting:

- 24 to 48 hours cleanse is when you go for an extended time in a fasting period and do not eat for 1 to 2 days.

- Using eating windows condenses your intake of macronutrients between a 4 to 7-hour window. The remainder of the time you are fasting.

- Skipping meals means you induce additional fasting times. Most people choose their skipped meal to be breakfast, but others choose lunch.

It is not recommended to go a straight 2 days without eating. You should begin by simply restriction you're eating windows. Many people, including myself, restrict eating from 5 to 11 pm. Others refer to their fasting windows with numbers, such as 19/5 or 21/3. This means 19 hours of fasting with a 5-hour eating window or 21 hours of fasting with a 3-hour eating window.

How Intermittent Fasting Works

The entire goal of intermittent fasting is to allow yourself to increase the food you consume at one time. Our bodies were made to consume a certain amount of food at once, so intermittent fasting is limiting our calorie intake, respectively.

Intermittent fasting by itself is naturally great for those that tend to overeat. Many of us forget to count the snacks we have throughout the day and still wonder why we pack on the weight. Your body will naturally adjust to the fasting method as you will find that you are not near as hunger as you used to be, which allows you to record and maintain values of nutrients you are consuming more efficiently.

3-Day Ketosis Boost – Applying Intermittent Fasting with the Keto Diet

To raise your ketone levels and kickstart your journey on the ketogenic diet, this 3-day fasting protocol developed by Tim Ferris is something that has worked for many people. This process helps you to get used to ketosis more quickly, so that you can transition with grace and stimulate further weight loss. If you are unable to go 3 days for the full fast, no worries. You will still illicit many benefits of fasting with the limitation of carb and protein consumption.

- *Thursday night*: Consume a keto dinner and make it the last meal of the day. Hit the hay like normal

- *Friday morning*: Walk within 30 minutes of waking up. Consume coffee or tea if you need to; it is best to limit your intake of caffeine. Bring at least 1 liter of water with you and add unrefined salt to it. Sip it as you walk to avoid cramps. Walk 3-4 throughout the day, sipping water as you need it the more walking, the better. This uses up your glycogen storage, which forces the body to move quickly into ketosis. The quicker ketosis takes over, better and less drained you will feel.

- *Friday afternoon/evening*: Consume MCT oil 2 to 3 times during the day. This gives you energy until your ketone levels are naturally elevated.

- *Saturday morning.* When you wake up, test your blood ketones. At 0.7mmol, proceed with fasting. Under? Take a walk and then re-test.

- *Saturday/Sunday.* Add MCT oil or coconut oil if you need a boost of energy. Incorporate salts in your water throughout the day

- *Sunday evening.* Break the fast with your favorite delicious ketogenic meal.

Chapter 11:
The 30-Day Ketogenic Diet Plan for Success

So far, you have learned a lot about what makes up the awesomeness of the Ketogenic Diet. Now, it is time for the tough part; creating a plan that you can truly stick to for more than just a few days. Switching your lifestyle from gorging on Krispy Kremes for breakfast and hitting up the nearest fast-food place for lunch to making your own meals and eating in can be very difficult. But if you are really dedicated to becoming healthier and losing that excess weight, you must have the willpower to give up the junk you're gueling your body with. Thankfully, this chapter will outline a meal plan to ensure your success as you utilize the Ketogenic Diet to lose weight and finally feel your best! Two main things before we get started:

- To increase calories, increase the amounts of fat you consume. Butter, macadamia nuts, olive and coconut oils are fantastic ways to increase fats. Drizzle, slather, and snack!

- To decrease calories, you need to consider what you need. More often than not, you will have to consume fewer proteins. This means you will need to keep in mind how big your meals will be. Decrease as you see fit.

WEEK ONE

The goal for week one is to start out simple; simplicity is key when beginning any new diet, let alone the keto. You don't want to make your body's transition any harder. Leftovers will become your best friend. It makes life easier and it will take some of the hassle from having to cook more often. Breakfast is a meal I personally always make extra for, so I don't have to rush around before work making something keto to begin my morning off right. It is much easier to grab pre-made items from the fridge.

You also need to keep an eye out for symptoms of the "keto flu", such as fogginess, fatique, headaches, etc. Ensure that you are consuming plenty of water and consuming salt. The ketogenic acts as a natrual diuretic, which means you will be peeing more than you are used to. Electrolytes are important! I suggest sprinkling a touch of salt into your water before drinking.

Breakfast: Week one's breakfasts should be easy, quick, and tasty. Also, pick recipes where you can make extra! Start day one on a weekend, so that you can make something for yourself the entire week ahead. Simplicity is key!

Lunch: Lunches during week one will be the same, simple and delicious. A simple salad paired with meat and drizzled with high in fat dressings are a great staple. You can also devour leftovers from dinner the night before as well.

Using canned meats? Make sure to read the labels and get options with the none or the least amount of additives!

Dinner: Week one's dinners will be a nice combo of meat piled high with leafy greens, such as spinach or broccoli. Again, remember that you want to consume high fat and moderate to small amounts of protein.

Dessert: Sorry. No sweets for the first two weeks. I have faith you can do it!

WEEK TWO

Week one will be over in a snap! You should have found it easy to keep track! Week two includes simple breakfasts, an intro to ketoproof coffee, and adding a decent mixture of heavy creams, butter, and coconut oils.

Breakfast: Week two we are going to change it up slightly for breakfast with your first round of ketoproof coffee! If you are not a coffee fan, try tea instead. Why ketoproof coffee?

Fat Loss. Plain and simple, the consumption of medium-chain triglycerides (MCT) has been shown to lead to greater losses in adipose tissue (fat tissue), in both animals and humans.

Fats! Eating fat has been shown to lead to greater amounts of energy, more efficient energy usage, and more effective weight loss. Not to mention, it's the main component of this diet.

More Energy. Studies have shown that the rapid rate of oxidation in MCFAs (Medium Chain Fatty Acids) leads to an increase in energy expenditure. Primarily, MCFAs are converted into ketones (our best friends), are absorbed differently in the body compared to regular oils and give us more overall energy.

If you have never tasted ketoproof coffee before, I would drink it slowly over the course of one to two hours. When you have a larger amount of coconut oil than you are used to, you will find yourself visiting the bathroom more often.

Lunch: Week two lunches are simple again, incorporating meat along with the previous night's dinners. Green veggies and high fat dressings will become your best friends!

Dinner: Dinners, to no surprise, will be simplistic too. High fat dressings, veggies, and meats will be the center of your last meal of the day.

Desserts: Remember, no dessert for this week either, but we'll be delving into that next week!

WEEK THREE

During week three you will be introducing your body to a small fasting period where you wil get your full on fasts during the morning hours and fast until dinner. This will give you many benefits and makes your eating schedule easier!

In a fasting state, our bodies can break down extra fat that's stored for the energy it needs. When we're in ketosis, our body already mimics a fasting state, being that we have little to no glucose in our bloodstream, so we use the fats in our bodies as energy. Intermittent fasting is using the same reasoning – instead of using the fats we are eating to gain energy, we are using our stored fat. That being said, you might think it's great – you can just fast and lose more weight. You have to take into account that later on, you will need to eat extra fat in order to keep out of a starvation mode state. There are a number of benefits shown that come from intermittent fasting:

- blood lipid levels
- longevity
- mental clarity

Don't do so hot with fasting yet? No biggie! Go back to week 1 and experiment as you see fit. You can eat what you want as long as it fits into your macros.

Breakfast: Just like during week two, you will be going hard on the fat intake. You should double your amount of ketoproof coffee or tea by doubling the amount of your fat of choice. This will be a lot of calories, which should keep you full until it is time to devour dinner!

Lunch: No lunch this week! The fats from your morning meal will keep you energized, satiated, and ready to eat once dinner time rolls around. Don't forget to drink water though!

Dinner: Dinner is staying the same as the previous weeks. Fats, veggies, and meats should be your staples! Also, it is time to mix in a few fun ketogenic carbs as well!

Dessert: Guess what?! You get to indulge in sweets this week! There are hundreds of great tasting treats to satisfy your sweet tooth.

WEEK FOUR

Week four will be a bit more challenging as you become stricter with your fasting routine. You had an entire week where you skipped lunch, but now we are going to forego both breakfast and lunch. Water will become your best friend! Don't forget to drink tons of liquids, ranging from flavored waters, tea, and coffee. Ignore your stomach's cries. If you cannot fast then you will need to go back to week two and try again. This is no big deal! Fasting is not easy and it takes time for your body to get used to this new concept. Just do the best you can!

Despite the negative stigmas of fasting, week four is my personal favorite because of how closely it resembles how I learned to eat on a daily basis. I set a 6-hour window for myself to eat within each day. After that, I wake up and until 5 in the evening I fast. I then open up my 'eating window' from 5 until 11 p.m. It will become fun for you because you can devour copious amounts of foods and be full until the next day! You also get to start experimenting more with dinner and desserts and you can snack as much as you want throughout your window.

Breakfast: Fasting! Black coffee if you're a caffeine addict like me. Tea, if you are not into the coffee so much. Tea can add great health benefits like coffee also. Some of the great benefits of green tea are:

Polyphenols – These function as antioxidants in your body. The most powerful antioxidant in green tea is Epigallocatechin gallate (EGCG), which has shown to be effective against fatigue.

- Improved Brain Function – Not only does green tea contain caffeine, but it also contains L-theanine, which is an amino acid. L-theanine increases your GABA activity, which improves anxiety, dopamine, and alpha waves.

- Increased Metabolic Rate – Green tea has been shown to improve your metabolic rate. In combination with the caffeine, this can lead up to 15% increased fat oxidization.

Lunch: Water, water, and more water. You don't get to eat lunch and you don't get to eat breakfast. So, make sure you keep yourself VERY hydrated. It's imperative here that you do a good job with your hydration. Remember – I recommend 4 liters a day.

Dinner: Lots and lots of food with dessert to cover the bases! Dinner is a fantastic time for me. I suggest breaking your fast with a small snack, then after 30-45 minutes eat to your heart's content. Normally I need 2 meals to get to my macros, and I think you'll need to do the same.

WEEK FIVE

Week five is where I depart from you and let you keep up your momentum on the ketogenic diet. You should have lots of leftovers frozen and waiting to be eaten! If this sample plan works great for you, then you are more than capable of creating your own meal plan that is specialized just for your lifestyle!

Creating Your Own Keto Meal Plan

- Think about what you eat and draft your own keto meal plan

- Check to see if your fats, proteins, and carbs match up to your body's weight.

- Research other keto diet plans to see how yours matches up. You do not want to jump into this diet head first.

- Revise any changes that need to be made. Improve upon anything that could be better.

- Talk with someone that has experiene with the ketogenic diet. They have even more tips from personal experience to share with you!

- Make final changes that you have to your diet plan and ensure that it is solid and matches up to your body's needs.

Chapter 12:
Delicious Ketogenic Recipes to Try!

Breakfast Recipes

Greek Egg Bake
Prep: 5 minutes

Cook time: 25 minutes

Makes 6 servings

Ingredients:
- ¼ C. sun dried tomatoes
- ½ C. feta cheese
- ½ tsp. oregano
- 1 C. chopped kale
- 12 eggs

Instructions:
1. Ensure your oven is preheated to 350 degrees.
2. With foil, line a baking sheet and spray with nonstick spray.

3. Whisk eggs and then stir in oregano, feta cheese, tomatoes, and kale.
4. Pour egg mixture into a sheet and bake 25 minutes.
5. Allow to cool for a few minutes before slicing.

Nutrition: 175 calories | 11g fat | 5g carbs | 15g protein

Blueberry Pancake Bites

Prep: 10 minutes

Cook time: 20-25 minutes

Makes 24 bites

Ingredients:
- ½ C. frozen blueberries
- 1/3 – ½ C. water
- ½ tsp. cinnamon
- ½ tsp. salt
- 1 tsp. baking powder
- ¼ C. melted ghee
- ½ C. coconut flour
- ½ tsp. vanilla extract
- 4 eggs

Instructions:
1. Ensure your oven is preheated to 325 degrees. Grease a muffin tin with butter and coconut oil spray.
2. Mix vanilla, sweetener, and eggs together until smooth.

3. Stir in cinnamon, salt, baking powder, melted ghee, and coconut flour, blending till smooth.
4. Add 1/3 cup of water to batter and blend once more. The batter should be thick.
5. Divide batter among muffin tin cups and add a few blueberries to each muffin.
6. Bake 20 to 25 minutes until set.
7. Allow cooling.

Can be kept in a cool place in an airtight container for 8-10 days. Can be frozen for 60-80 days.

Nutrition: 188 calories | 13g fat | 7.5g carbs | 6g protein

Low Carb Breakfast Pizza

Prep: 10 minutes

Cook time: 30 minutes

Makes 8 servings

Ingredients:
- ¼ tsp. pepper
- ½ C. heavy cream
- ½ tsp. salt
- 1 C. shredded cheese of choice
- 12 eggs
- 2 C. sliced peppers
- 8 ounces of sausage

Instructions:
1. Ensure your oven is preheated to 350 degrees.
2. Microwave peppers for 3 minutes.
3. In a cast iron skillet, brown sausage. Set to the side.
4. Mix pepper, salt, cream, and eggs together and place in skillet.
5. Cook 5 minutes till the sides begin to become firm.
6. Place skillet in over and back 15 minutes. Remove from oven.

7. Add cheese, peppers, and sausage to skillet and place under broiler for 3 minutes.
8. Allow to sit for 5 minutes to cool. Devour right away or split between meal prep containers.

Can be refrigerated for 5 days or frozen for 60 days.

Nutrition: 307 calories | 16g fat | 7g carbs | 19g protein

Banana Strawberry Baked Oatmeal

Prep: 10 minutes

Cook time: 35-40 minutes

Makes 8 servings

Ingredients:
- ¼ C. pure maple syrup
- ½ tsp. salt
- 1 ½ C. chopped strawberries + more to serve
- 1 tsp. baking powder
- 1 tsp. cinnamon
- 2 eggs
- 2 tsp. vanilla extract
- 3 C. almond milk
- 3 mashed/ripe bananas
- 4 C. old-fashioned oats

Instructions:
1. Ensure your oven is preheated to 350 degrees. Grease a baking dish.
2. Whisk salt, baking powder, cinnamon, vanilla, maple syrup, milk, eggs, and banana together well.

3. Mix in oats. Gently fold in strawberries.
4. Pour mixture onto the prepared dish.
   Bake 35-40 minutes till oatmeal sets.
5. Allow to sit 5 minutes before serving. Serve topped with more chopped strawberries.

Leftovers can be refrigerated for 3 days. Simply reheat oatmeal with a bit of almond milk and top with desired fruit if you so choose.

Nutrition: 154 calories | 16g fat | 6g carbs | 14g protein

Turkey Chorizo Breakfast Sandwich

Prep: 20 minutes

Cook time: 10 minutes

Makes 1 serving

Ingredients:
Turkey Chorizo:

- ¼ tsp. cayenne pepper
- ¼ tsp. cinnamon
- ¼ tsp. dried thyme
- ¼ tsp. onion powder
- ¼ tsp. pepper
- ½ tsp. dried oregano
- 1 tbsp. cumin
- 1 tbsp. paprika
- 1 tsp. coriander
- 1 tsp. fennel seeds
- 1 tsp. garlic powder
- 1 tsp. sea salt

- 1/8 tsp. ground cloves
- 1-pound lean ground turkey breast

Breakfast Sandwich:
- ¼ avocado
- 1 cooked turkey chorizo patty
- 1 egg
- 1 whole wheat English muffin

Instructions:
1. TO make chorizo: Add turkey and spices to a bowl and mix well with hands. Create 16 even-sized portions and make them into ¼-inch patties.
2. Cook chorizo patties in a greased skillet till patties turn brown.
3. To make sandwich: Spray a skillet and add egg. Cook to your preference.
4. Toast your English muffin.
5. Serve muffin topped with one chorizo patty, eggs, and avocado.

Nutrition: 203 calories | 11g fat | 8g carbs | 29g protein

Lunch Recipes

Mediterranean Salad

Prep: 5 minutes

Cook: 10 minutes

Total: 15 minutes

Servings: 2

Ingredients:
- 1 C. cooked whole-grain couscous
- 1 tbsp. olive oil
- 2 ounces crumbles feta cheese
- 4-5 slices artichoke hearts marinated in olive oil
- 6-10 cherry tomatoes
- Juice of ½ a lemon
- Sea salt
- Sprinkle of dried basil, oregano, and parsley

Instructions:
1. Mix all liquid ingredients together to create a type of dressing.

2. Pour dressing into the bottom of the jar. Then add other ingredients to jar as you see fit.

Refrigerate for up to 3 days.

Nutrition: 201 calories | 4g fat | 2g carbs | 13g protein

Chipotle Turkey and Sweet Potato Chili

Prep: 5 minutes

Cook: 20 minutes

Total: 25 minutes

Servings: 4

Ingredients:

- ¼ - ½ tsp. ground chipotle powder
- 1 C. diced onion
- 1 sweet potato
- 1 tbsp. coconut oil
- 1 tsp. cumin
- 1 tsp. dried oregano
- 1-pound ground turkey
- 2 C. chicken broth
- 2 tsp. chili powder
- 28-ounces fire roasted tomatoes
- Pepper and salt

Instructions:

1. Warm up coconut oil over intermediate-extreme warmth.
2. Once the oil begins to simmer, place the turkey in pan. Cook 5 minutes, breaking up as it cooks.
3. Toss in garlic and onions, cooking 8-10 minutes till onions turn translucent.
4. Turn warmth up to high. Pour in broth, sweet potato, and tomatoes, along with seasonings. Bring the mixture up to boiling point.
5. Turn down heat to medium and allow to simmer for 10-15 minutes uncovered. The longer you allow to simmer, the bigger the flavor.

Nutrition: 423 calories | 18g fat | 14g carbs | 28g protein

Avocado Bacon Garlic Burger

Prep: 15 minutes

Cook: 8-10 minutes

Total: 30 minutes

Servings: 4

Ingredients:
- ½ tsp. pepper
- 1 C. chopped basil
- 1 tsp. salt
- 1-pound grass-fed lean ground beef
- 2 eggs
- 3 minced cloves garlic

Toppings:
- 1 avocado
- 16 pieces of bacon cooked
- 4 slices red onion

Instructions:
1. Mix all hamburger components till well incorporated.

2. Divide meat into four patties.
3. Warm up olive oil in a pan.
4. Place patties in pan, grilling 4 minutes per side.
5. Make burgers with avocado as the bun and other desired toppings.

Nutrition: 189 calories | 22g fat | 9g carbs | 27g protein

Zucchini Lasagna

Prep: 10-15 minutes

Cook: 25 minutes

Total: 40 minutes

Servings: 4-6

Ingredients:
- ¼ C. minced parsley
- ½ C. diced onion
- ½ pound lean ground turkey
- ½ tbsp. Italian seasoning
- ½ tbsp. minced garlic
- ½ tsp. oregano
- 1 C. part-skim mozzarella cheese
- 1 egg yolk
- 1 tbsp. olive oil
- 2 tsp. salt
- 2 zucchinis
- 4 tsp. parmesan cheese

- 6 tbsp. canned tomato sauce
- 6 tbsp. crushed tomatoes
- 8 ounces low-fat ricotta cheese

Instructions:
1. Ensure oven is preheated to 350 degrees.
2. Slice zucchinis 1/8" thick and sprinkle with 1 ½ tsp. salt.
3. Bake 15-25 minutes till water is released from edges.
4. Lay zucchini out on paper towels. Reduce oven temp to 325 degrees.
5. Warm olive oil in a pan, then pour turkey, garlic and onion, cooking meat till cooked through. Season with seasonings. Set aside.
6. Mix crushed tomatoes and tomato sauce together. Season with salt and pepper.
7. Mix pepper, salt, egg, and ricotta together as well.
8. Layer half of sauce between 4 jars. Then layer turkey, zucchini noodles and other ingredients. Parsley, mozzarella should go on top. Seal jars well.

Can be refrigerated for 3 days.

Nutrition: 114 calories | 9g fat | 3g carbs | 8g protein

Mashed Parmesan and Chive Cauliflower

Prep: 10 minutes

Cook: 20 minutes

Total: 30 minutes

Makes 6 servings

Ingredients:
- ¼ C. chopped chives
- ¼ C. grated Parmesan cheese
- 2 C. chicken broth
- 2 heads of cauliflower cored/cut into florets

Instructions:
1. Pour cauliflower florets and chicken broth into a pot and heat to boiling.
2. Reduce heat and cover lid. Cook 15 to 20 minutes until cauliflower becomes tender.
3. With a slotted spoon, remove cauliflower into a food processor and puree until smooth.
4. Pour cauliflower puree into a serving bowl and stir Parmesan cheese and chives in, seasoning with pepper and salt to achieve desired taste.

Nutrition: 297 calories | 13g fat | 4g carbs | 10g protein

Dinner Recipes

Instant Pot Lamb Shanks

Prep: 10 minutes

Cook: 50 minutes

Total: 1 hour

Servings: 3-4

Ingredients:

- ¼ C. minced Italian parsley
- 1 C. bone broth
- 1 chopped onion
- 1 tbsp. balsamic vinegar
- 1 tbsp. tomato paste
- 1 tsp. red boat fish sauce
- 1-pound ripe Roma tomatoes
- 2 chopped carrots
- 2 chopped celery stalks
- 2 tbsp. ghee

- 3 pounds lamb shanks
- 3 smashed/peeled garlic cloves
- Pepper and salt

Instructions:
1. Season with shanks with pepper and salt.
2. Press SAUTE on instant pot, melt tablespoon ghee. Place shanks into pot and sear on all sides 8-10 minutes.
3. As lamb browns chop up veggies. Take out lamb from pot.
4. Lower heat and add remaining ghee. Then add onion, celery, and carrots to the pot, seasoning with pepper and salt.
5. Add tomato paste and garlic cloves, stirring at least 60 seconds.
6. Place shanks back into the pot along with tomatoes.
7. Pour balsamic vinegar, fish sauce, and bone broth into the pot.
8. Lock lid. Press MANUAL and set to cook 50 minutes. Perform natural release.
9. Remove shanks to plate and top with sauce.

Nutrition: 338 calories | 32g fat | 11g carbs | 41g protein

Garlic Pork and Kale

Prep: 10 minutes

Cook: 40 minutes

Total: 1 hour

Servings: 4-6

Ingredients:
- 1 tbsp. red wine vinegar
- 1 tsp. minced rosemary
- 20-25 whole garlic cloves
- 2 sprigs of thyme
- 1 chopped yellow onion
- 2 tbsp. olive oil
- 2 ½ pound boneless pork shoulder (cut into 1 ½-inch chunks)
- 2/3 C. chicken broth
- 2/3 C. dry red wine

Instructions:
1. Season pork liberally with pepper and salt.

2. Press SAUTE on instant pot and heat up olive oil. Working in batches, sear pork till browned. Remove with slotted spoon. Discard fat from instant pot.
3. Add thyme and onion to instant pot, sautéing 5 minutes. Then add rosemary and garlic, cooking 60 seconds.
4. Pour wine in, using a wooden spoon to deglaze the bits from bottom of the pot.
5. Pour in broth and add pork back in. Combine.
6. Lock lid. Press MANUAL to cook 40 minutes. Perform quick release.
7. Stir in kale. Press HIGH PRESSURE to cook another 10 minutes. Perform another quick release.
8. Kale and pork should be nice and tender.

You can freeze up to 3 months.

Nutrition: 437 calories | 31g fat | 12g carbs | 47g protein

Beef and Broccoli

Prep: 20 minutes

Cook: 40 minutes

Total: 1 hour

Servings: 4-6

Ingredients:
- ¼ tsp. fresh ginger
- 1 tbsp. cooking oil
- 10 to 12-ounce flank steak or sirloin
- 2 minced cloves garlic
- 3 ½ C. broccoli florets
- Water

Marinade:
- ¼ tsp. dark soy sauce
- ½ tsp. sesame oil
- 1 tsp. cornstarch
- 1 tsp. low-sodium soy sauce
- 1/8 tsp. pepper

Sauce:

- ¼ tsp. dark soy sauce
- ½ tsp. dry sherry
- 1 ½ tbsp. oyster flavored sauce
- 1 ½ tsp. low-sodium soy sauce
- 1 tsp. toasted sesame oil
- 1/3 C. cold water
- 2 tsp. cornstarch
- 2 tsp. sugar

Instructions:
1. Mix all marinade ingredients together. Add beef slices and let sit at least 10 minutes.
2. Blanch broccoli.
3. Combine all sauce ingredients together.
4. Warm oil in a pan or wok. Add beef in a single layer to sear. Pour garlic and continue cooking meat till cooked through. Pour sauce in, constantly stirring till it becomes thickened. Add more water to thin it out if needed. Add broccoli and stir everything well to coat. Season with pepper and salt if desired.
5. Sprinkle sesame seeds and chopped onions if desired.

6. Divide among containers.

Nutrition: 259 calories | 9g fat | 12g carbs | 28g protein

Chipotle Turkey and Sweet Potato Chili

Prep: 5 minutes

Cook: 20 minutes

Total: 25 minutes

Servings: 4

Ingredients:
- ¼ - ½ tsp. ground chipotle powder
- 1 C. diced onion
- 1 sweet potato
- 1 tbsp. coconut oil
- 1 tsp. cumin
- 1 tsp. dried oregano
- 1-pound ground turkey
- 2 C. chicken broth
- 2 tsp. chili powder
- 28-ounces fire roasted tomatoes
- 3 minced cloves garlic
- Pepper and salt

Instructions:
1. Warm up coconut oil over intermediate-extreme warmth.
2. Once the oil begins to simmer, place the turkey in pan. Cook 5 minutes, breaking up as it cooks.
3. Toss in garlic and onions, cooking 8-10 minutes till onions turn translucent.
4. Turn warmth up to high. Pour in broth, sweet potato, and tomatoes, along with seasonings. Bring the mixture up to boiling point.
5. Turn down heat to medium and allow to simmer for 10-15 minutes uncovered. The longer you allow to simmer, the bigger the flavor.

Refrigerate for 7 days and freeze for up to 6 months.

Nutrition: 423 calories | 18g fat | 14g carbs | 28g protein

Keto Meatballs

Prep: 15 minutes

Cook: 15 minutes

Total: 30 minutes

Servings: 10-12

Ingredients:
- ¼ tsp. dried oregano
- ¼ tsp. garlic powder
- ¼ tsp. pepper
- ½ C. almond flour
- ¾ C. grated parmesan cheese
- 1 ½ pounds ground beef
- 1 tsp. dried onion flakes
- 1 tsp. salt
- 1/3 C. warm water
- 2 eggs
- 2 tbsp. chopped parsley
- 1 tsp. olive oil

- 3 C. keto marinara sauce

Instructions:
1. In a bowl, mix all meatball components with your hands.
2. Form mixture into 2" balls.
3. With olive oil, coat your instant pot.
4. Brown meatballs in a skillet.
5. Layer meatballs and marinara into your instant pot.
6. Set to MANUAL and push LOW to cook 10 minutes.
7. Perform a quick release.
8. Serve with zoodles!

Nutrition: 212 calories | 13g fat | 8g carbs | 18g protein

Dessert Recipes

Walnut Orange Chocolate Bombs

Prep: 15 minutes

Freeze: 1 to 3 hours

Total: 3.5 hours

Servings: 8

Ingredients:

- ¼ C. extra virgin coconut oil
- ½-1 tbsp. orange peel or orange extract
- 1 ¾ C. chopped walnuts
- 1 tsp. cinnamon
- 10-15 drops stevia
- 125g 85% cocoa dark chocolate

Instructions:

1. Melt chocolate with your choice of method.
2. Add cinnamon and coconut oil. Sweeten mixture with stevia.
3. Pour in fresh orange peel and chopped walnuts.
4. In a muffin tin or in candy cups, spoon in mixture.

5. Place into the fridge for 1-3 hours until mixture is solid.

Nutrition: 87 calories | 9g fat | 2g carbs | 2g protein

Peanut Butter Chocolate Bombs

Prep: 30 minutes

Total: 30 hours

Servings: 6

Ingredients:
- ¼ C. chopped walnuts
- ½ C. butter or coconut oil
- ½ C. plain or chunky natural peanut butter
- ½ tsp. vanilla extract
- 1 C. sweetener of choice
- 1/3 C. cocoa powder
- 1/3 C. vanilla whey powder
- 2 oz. softened cream cheese
- Dash of salt

Instructions:
1. Line a 5x7 dish with parchment paper, ensuring there is an overhang of paper of two sides to aid in removal later. Spread melted butter over paper as well.

2. In a saucepan over low heat, melt butter and peanut butter together, combining well.
3. In another bowl, beat cream cheese until it soft and proceed to beat in peanut butter until mixture is smooth.
4. Add in sugar substitute and vanilla.
5. Mix together salt, cocoa powder, and protein powder in a separate bowl, sifting dry ingredients into wet ones until smooth in texture. Stir in nuts.
6. Spread fudge mixture into prepared pan, placing in the freezer to harden.
7. Remove and cut into squares. Store in the chilled area before serving.

Nutrition: 211 calories | 18g fat | 2g carbs | 4g protein

Chocolate Coconut Bites

Prep: 5 minutes

Cook: 0 minutes

Total: 5-10 minutes

Servings: 8+

Ingredients:

- ½ C. pecans
- ½ C. shredded unsweetened coconut flakes
- 1 tbsp. almond milk
- 1 tbsp. chia seeds
- 1 tbsp. cocoa powder
- 1 tbsp. collagen peptides
- 1 tbsp. liquid coconut oil
- 2 tbsp. hemp seeds
- 8 dates pitted
- Extra coconut flakes (optional)

Instructions:

1. Blend all recipe components within a food processor till well incorporated.
2. Roll mixture into 1" balls. Roll in additional coconut flakes if you so choose.

Freeze for up to 60 days.

Nutrition: 71 calories | 16g fat | 8g carbs | 7g protein

Oatmeal Energy Bites

Prep: 5 minutes

Freeze: 60 minutes

Total: 1 hour

Servings: 8

Ingredients:

- ¼ C. ground flax seed
- ½ C. chocolate chips
- ½ C. almond butter
- 1 C. rolled oats
- 1/3 C. raw honey

Instructions:
1. Mix all recipe components together.
2. Roll out teaspoon sized balls onto a tray lined with parchment paper.
3. Freeze balls for 1 hour.

Freeze for up to 1 month.

Nutrition: 71 calories | 16g fat | 5g carbs | 7g protein

Smoothie Recipes

Green Early Morning Smoothie
Prep: 10 minutes

Ingredients:
- 1 ½ C. water
- 4 C. fresh kale
- ½ a whole lemon
- ½ cucumber

Instructions:
1. Add avocado, lemon, and cucumber to your blender.
2. Pack the remaining portion of the blender with kale and add water.
3. Pulse until well incorporated and smooth.

Nutrition: 51 calories | 2g fat | 0g carbs | 2g protein

Chocolate Almond Smoothie

Prep: 10 minutes

Ingredients:
- ¼ C. ice
- 1 C. almond milk
- 1 scoop of Stevia
- 1 tbsp. cacao powder
- 2 tbsp. avocado

Instructions:
1. Add all ingredients to your blender.
2. Pulse until smooth and creamy.

Nutrition: 92 calories | 9g fat | 2g carbs | 6g protein

Blueberry Power Smoothie

Prep: 10 minutes

Ingredients:

- ¼ C. 2% plain Greek yogurt
- ½ C. fresh or frozen strawberries or blueberries
- ½ tsp. pure vanilla
- 1 C. coconut milk
- 1 tbsp. gelatin
- 1 tbsp. virgin coconut oil
- 3 servings of Stevia
- 5 ice cubes

Instructions:

1. Place all ingredients into your blender.
2. Pulse until frozen fruit and ice are well incorporated and the mixture is smooth.

Nutrition: 147 calories | 17g fat | 6g carbs | 9g protein

Chapter 13:
Ketogenic Tips and Tricks

Your main goal when you are maintaining your lifestyle on the Ketogenic Diet is keeping your body within a stable state of ketosis. Even though this sounds challenging, and it can be for some dieters, there are many things you can do to keep your ketosis levels at peak performance.

Staying hydrated every day is something you should already be doing but many people fail to drink enough water. When you first get out of bed, challenge yourself to drink 32-ounces of water and then do your best to consume another 32 to 48-ounces before the noon hour. You should strive to consume at least half of your weight in ounces of water daily to ensure you are fully hydrated. If you are not used to drinking this much water each day, you are not alone; many individuals don't. Do your best to consume near the amounts until you build your tolerance up for it.

Practice intermittent fasting to start reducing your carb intake a few days before starting to implement the ketogenic diet. To do this successfully, you should break your day down into two phases:

- The building phase is the amount of time between your first and last meal.

- The cleaning phase is the amount of time between your last and first meal.

To ensure maximum success, you should start with a cleaning phase of 12 to 16 hours paired with a building phase of 8 to 12 hours. This will help the body to adapt over time, which enables you to decrease your building phase to 4 to 6 hours and increase your cleaning phase to 18 to 20 hours. This helps to maintain your levels of ketosis much easier.

Consume good salts to reduce your consumption of sodium. When you start a diet low in carbohydrate consumptions, your insulin levels will naturally decrease as your kidneys excrete high levels of sodium. This lowers the ratio of potassium and sodium in your body, which means you will crave sodium more. Here are some healthy ways to ensure your body isn't deficient in sodium levels:

- Add ¼ teaspoon of pink salt to glasses of water

- Be generous with the amount of pink salt you add to food

- Consume pumpkin seeds or macadamia nuts as a snack

- Drink organic broth off and on throughout the day

- Eat cucumbers or celery, both have natural sodium

Regular exercise helps to activate glucose molecules, also known as GLUT-4, that communicates information to different areas of your body and then back to the tissues of the liver and muscles. This specific glucose receptor eliminates sugar from the blood stream and uses it as glycogen in the liver and muscles. Therefore, daily exercise doubles the levels of these crucial proteins in your liver and muscles.

Improve the mobility of your bowels so that ketosis can do its job easier. One of the downfalls of starting the ketogenic diet is struggling with bouts of constipation. Thankfully, there are some ways to regulate your bowels without getting off track:

- Consume fermented foods, such as sauerkraut, kimchi, coconut water, etc.

- Take supplements such as magnesium.

- Drink at least one serving of green tea per day to increase your calcium and potassium levels.

Don't consume too much protein even though it has been strongly stated that the consumption of proteins is recommended as it is required by the ketogenic diet, some people do not know a proper balance and eat too much protein. If you consume too much, your body will change all those amino acids into glucose through the process known as gluconeogenesis. You will probably have to play with the amounts of protein you eat because some people need more or less than others.

You should aim for 1 gram of protein per kilogram of body weight. For example, if you weigh 160 pounds that comes out to 2.2 pound per kilogram, which equals about 73 grams of protein. It is best to consume 2-3 servings of 15-50 grams of protein per meal.

Choose the carbs you consume wisely even though the ketogenic diet recommends to stay far away from carbs, it is in your best interest to at least consume some good types of carbohydrates, such as starchy veggies and fruits such as limes, lemon, apples, and berries These are especially good if combined within a green protein shake.

Utilize MCT oil when you can while on the ketogenic diet, the use of high-quality medium chain triglyceride (MCT) is crucial in maintaining the state of ketosis. This is because this oil allows those that consume it to eat more carbs/proteins and still maintain a good level for ketosis. You can not only cook with this oil but add it to coffee, tea, green drinks, protein shakes and more!

Keep stress to a minimum which is easier said than done, I know. But daily stress will inhibit the process of ketosis to the point of being non-existent. If you are under constant chronic stress, then now may not be the time to undergo the ketogenic diet, but rather an anti-inflammatory, lower carb diet instead.

Learn ways to improve the quality of sleep if you are not receiving adequate amounts of rest, this is another aspect that can lead to a rise in stress hormones. Ensure that you catch your rest in a dark room that you feel comfortable in. It is recommended to receive around 7-9 hours of sleep per night. The more stressed you are, the more sleep you need. Ensure that you are sleeping in a room that is no warmer than 65-70 degrees.

Consume so ghee, ghee is a grand substitute for butter and is highly recommended on the ketogenic diet. You can use it as normally as you utilize butter.

Take Omega-3's, it is vital that you consume or take Omega-3 vitamins. You should have higher levels of Omega 3's than Omega 6's in your diet. Eating all that oil will cause you harm if your Omegas are not properly balanced.

Avoid alcohol, I know, this doesn't sound that fun. But the consumption of alcohol quite literally puts an abrupt stop to your weight loss. Which is worth it: that glass of wine or being able to fit into those skinnier pants?

Lemon water is your friend, not only is it tasty and pretty darn refreshing, but lemon water balances out your pH levels in your body, creating a better environment for ketosis to properly thrive.

Avoid "sugar-free" products, even though it sounds better for you, try to avoid products that say "sugar-free" or "light" because these more than likely have more cars than their original counterparts.

Avoid low-fat, while on the ketogenic diet, you should steer clear and not waste your precious time with anything that is low in fat. You need to have high percentages of fat in your diet in order to maintain an adequate and healthy balance. Otherwise, the protein you consume may be converted into sugars too.

Conclusion

Life is much more than becoming a slave to your taste buds; to really live you need the energy and the body to enjoy it to its fullest potential! And the Ketogenic Diet is one of the best avenues to get your diet in check and feel the best you have in years. I hope that this book was not only informative and valuable, but I hope it also brought a spark of inspiration to begin making changes to how you fuel your body and mind starting *today*. Why put off tomorrow what you can start right now?!

As you are aware, change of any kind is challenging, let alone the habits you have created when it comes to what you eat. Taking baby steps, no matter how tiny, will be one of the biggest things that ensures your success and enables you to stick to the Ketogenic Diet for weeks to come. The next step you need to take once you close this book is to accept that you need to change your habits; you will never have the willpower to change anything in life unless you unmask your negative daily habits. Yes, this includes sneaking food from the fridge at midnight and hitting up the convenience store for a quick bite and sugary beverage.

Change is hard, but I know you can do it! After all, you found this book and red it all the way to this point! That already says something about your character! Search online and reference back to the shopping list chapter as well as the sample meal plans to get started creating your plan for the Ketogenic journey you are about to encounter!

I wish you the best of luck as you and your taste buds discover that fresh, fattier foods taste much better than that of other diets and that you can do this!

If you find this book helpful in anyway a review to support my endeavors is much appreciated.

www.ingramcontent.com/pod-product-compliance
Lightning Source LLC
Chambersburg PA
CBHW020257030426
42336CB00010B/804